DATE DUE

MAR 0 6 1992	
3-25-96 ILL	
ILL 7913625	2/13/99
FEB 1 6 1999	

HANDBOOK OF VERTIGO

HANDBOOK OF VERTIGO

Michael E. Glasscock III, M.D., F.A.C.S.
Roberto A. Cueva, M.D.
Britt A. Thedinger, M.D.

The Otology Group, P.C.
Nashville, Tennessee

Raven Press New York

Raven Press, Ltd., 1185 Avenue of the Americas, New York, New York 10036

Made in the United States of America.

Library of Congress Cataloging-in-Publication Data

Glasscock, Michael E., 1933–
    Handbook of vertigo / Michael E. Glasscock III, Roberto A. Cueva, Britt A. Thedinger.
        p.   cm.
    Includes bibliographical references.
    Includes index.
    ISBN 0-88167-688-8
    1. Vestibular apparatus—Diseases—Handbooks, manuals, etc.
2. Vertigo—Handbooks, manuals, etc.   I. Cueva, Roberto A.
II Thedinger, Britt A.   III. Title.
    [DNLM: 1. Vertigo—handbooks.   WV 39 G549h]
RF260.G53   1990
617.8'82—dc20
DNLM/DLC
for Library of Congress   90-8765
                                                                   CIP

The material contained in this volume was submitted as previously unpublished material, except in the instances in which credit has been given to the source from which some of the illustrative material was derived.

Great care has been taken to maintain the accuracy of the information contained in the volume. However, neither Raven Press nor the editors can be held responsible for errors or for any consequences arising from the use of the information contained herein.

Materials appearing in this book prepared by individuals as part of their official duties as U.S. Government employees are not covered by the above-mentioned copyright.

9 8 7 6 5 4 3 2 1

Preface

This handbook concerns the vestibular system and how it functions. It is directed toward medical students and residents and is designed as a general review of the subject rather than as a reference source. The authors cover the subject in a thorough, yet abbreviated manner and include: (1) anatomy and physiology, (2) common vestibular disorders, (3) diagnostic studies, and (4) case histories. A comprehensive reference list has been compiled to stimulate a more extensive study of the vestibular system.

Michael E. Glasscock, III

Contents

HANDBOOK OF VERTIGO

1

Anatomy and Physiology of the Vestibular System

Anatomy
Physiology
Summary
Suggested Reading

This chapter focuses on the basic anatomy and physiology of the vestibular system. The relationship between the endolymphatic and perilymphatic chambers is discussed. The results of endolymphatic movement in the semicircular canals is outlined to encourage an understanding with relationship to vestibular testing. Basic theoretic principles regarding the mechanism of function for the utricular macula are reviewed. Current difficulties in understanding the central integration of compiled balance information are expressed.

ANATOMY

The peripheral vestibular system is made up of the three semicircular canals (superior, lateral, and posterior), the saccule, and the utricle. The semicircular canals are oriented at perpendicular axes to each other, approximating the planes of three-dimensional space. The utricle and saccule occupy the elliptical and spherical recesses, respectively, in the main chamber of the bony vestibule (Fig. 1). Within the bony framework of the vestibule are found the two compartments of the membranous labyrinth, the endolymphatic and perilymphatic spaces. The endolymphatic portion of the membranous vestibule contains the sensory neuroepithelium critical to ves-

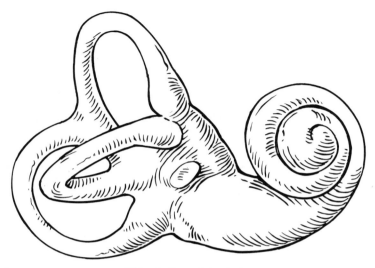

FIG. 1. Bony labyrinth.

tibular function. These sensory structures are made up of the cristae in the ampullae of the semicircular canals, and the maculae, which lie in the saccule and utricle.

The components of the endolymphatic chamber are the three semicircular canals, the utricle, the saccule, and the scala media of the cochlea, as well as the endolymphatic duct and sac (Fig. 2). The ampullae of the superior and lateral canals have wide open communications with the utricle in the region of the utricular macula. The posterior semicircular canal has its ampullary connection with the utricle in its inferior aspect, somewhat distanced from the macula. The endolymph in these canals flows freely into the utricular space. The nonampullated ends of the superior and posterior semicircular canals join to form the common crus prior to entering the utricle. The nonampullated end of the lateral canal has its own entrance into the utricle. In contrast to the widely patent communications shared between the utricle and semicircular canals, the utricle is connected to the saccule by a sliver-thin utriculo–endolymphatic duct. It is along this narrow connection between utricle and saccule that the endolymphatic duct, leading to the endolymphatic sac, communicates with the rest of the endolymphatic chamber. The saccule in

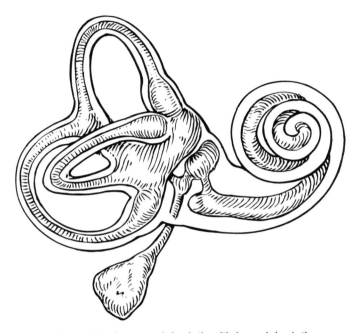

FIG. 2. Membranous labyrinth with bony labyrinth.

turn connects with the cul-de-sac of the cochlear duct. The cochlear duct in its spiral course through the cochlea is also known as the scala media.

The perilymphatic chamber virtually surrounds the endolymphatic chambers. In the vestibular portion of the labyrinth it plays a more passive role, whereas in the cochlea it is the movement of perilymph in the scala tympani that vibrates the basement membrane of the organ of Corti. This vibration stimulates the hair cells embedded in the tectorial membrane. The perilymphatic spaces parallel the endolymphatic spaces in the semicircular canals and main body of the vestibule. In the cochlea the perilymphatic spaces are made up of the scala tympani and scala vestibuli.

The peripheral vestibular system is connected to the central nervous system via the superior and inferior vestibular branches of the eighth cranial nerve. Scarpa's ganglion (the vestibular ganglion) is made up of the bodies of bipolar cells, and rests in the lateral aspect of the internal auditory canal. Its short peripheral processes synapse with the receptor cells of the cristae and maculae. The long central processes form the vestibular nerve, which synapses with the vestibular nuclei and cerebellum. The superior vestibular nerve innervates the derivatives of the embryologic pars superioris, that is, the cristae of the superior and lateral semicircular canals and the utricular macula. There is also a small branch that provides some innervation to the saccular macula. The inferior vestibular nerve innervates the pars inferioris derivatives, namely, the crista of the posterior semicircular canal and the saccular macula (Fig. 3). An in-depth discussion of the central component of the vestibular system, specifically the four vestibular nuclei, their interconnections, and their connections to the peripheral system and brain is beyond the scope of this book. Suffice it to say that there is topographical organization of the

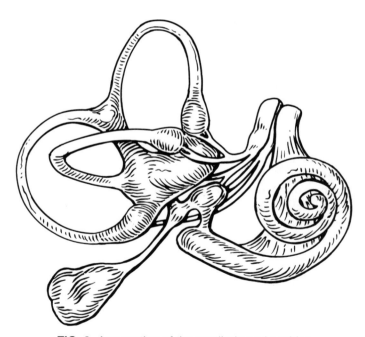

FIG. 3. Innervation of the vestibule and cochlea.

neuronal connections from the end organ to the level of the vestibular nuclei and beyond.

PHYSIOLOGY

The function of the vestibular system is to maintain the equilibrium of the individual with relationship to movement and Earth's gravity. The arrangement of the semicircular canals and otolithic organs (utricle and saccule) accomplishes these goals by converting the mechanical energy of movement, or shift in position relative to gravity, to electrical inputs processed by the brain.

At rest, the paired vestibular end organs provide a baseline of tonic discharge relayed to the vestibular nuclei and cerebellum. If this symmetric tonic discharge is suddenly altered (in most vestibular dysfunctions this means a unilateral reduction in firing) then the imbalanced input received by the central nervous system is perceived as continuous head motion. The clinical manifestation of this imbalance is vertigo, nystagmus, and the autonomic responses of nausea and vomiting.

Quickly realizing that the organism cannot survive in such a chaotic state, the central nervous system takes emergency measures in the form of "cerebellar clamp." This is a short-term inhibitory feedback from the cerebellum to the vestibular nuclei, causing a decrease in the perceived imbalance until the cortex and higher centers can adapt to the altered baseline tonic discharge provided by the diseased vestibular end organ. The higher centers of the central nervous system are very efficient at adapting to the altered function and will utilize the other sensory modalities important to equilibrium to override the "erroneous information" being delivered by the vestibular system. These other sensory modalities include: visual input, somatosensory data, and proprioceptive information.

To understand the significance of vestibular testing results, comprehension of how the peripheral vestibular end organ does its job is essential. Rotational head movement in three-dimensional space is thought to be primarily sensed by the semicircular canals in the form of rotational acceleration. For example, when the head (tilted forward 30° to place the lateral semicircular canal parallel to the ground) turns to the right, the rotational acceleration generated is sensed primarily by the lateral semicircular canals.

The endolymph in the horizontal semicircular canal of the right ear will remain stationary relative to the moving head due to the influence of inertia. This will cause a relative utriculopetal (toward the utricle) movement of endolymph within the canal, which in turn causes an increase in the firing rate of the neuroepithelium. The endolymph in the left semicircular canal, operating under the same influences, experiences a relative utriculofugal (away from the utricle) movement, causing a decrease in the firing rate of the neuroepithelium on the left. The input from the right and left end organs is then sent to their respective vestibular nuclei and the cerebellum. Centrally the balanced signal of increased firing on the right combined with decreased firing on the left tells the brain that the head is turning to the right.

The relationship between this pattern of neural firing and the reactions seen during caloric testing are classically explained as follows. Cold water caloric testing in the supine position causes a relative increase in the density of the endolymph in the lateral semicircular canal. In the supine position (head tilted back 60°) the lateral canal is nearly in the vertical plane. This increase in endolymph density causes a slight shift in the endolymph toward gravity, resulting in utriculofugal movement of endolymph, therefore decreasing neural firing on the tested side. The dominant normal firing of the opposite ear drives the eyes toward the tested ear via the vestibular input to the optokinetic reflex. This is the slow phase of nystagmus. The more noticeable fast phase is the compensatory saccade generated by higher centers trying to return the eyes to primary gaze. Primary gaze directs the eyes straight ahead with reference to the head. Hence, cold water stimulation of an ear will cause a nystagmus that beats (fast-phase nystagmus) to the opposite ear. The converse is true of warm water stimulation. Warm water causes a relative decrease in the endolymphatic density. This warmed endolymph rises in the lateral canal, resulting in an utriculopetal flow of endolymph. This flow results in increased firing from the tested ear, which drives the eyes to look to away from the tested ear. The compensatory saccade, fast-phase nystagmus, is then in the direction of the tested ear, and is interpreted as nystagmus beating to the tested ear. This is the basis for the mnemonic COWS (Cold–Opposite/Warm–Same). This "convection theory" of caloric stimulation has been challenged by recent studies on caloric testing done in space under weightless conditions. These most recent studies suggest a direct temperature effect on the vestibular end organ as, at least, a contributing factor in the observed clinical findings.

This pattern of neuroepithelial response relative to endolymphatic movement is reversed for the superior and posterior semicircular canals, that is, utriculopetal movement of endolymph causes a reduction in neural firing, while utriculofugal endolymphatic movement causes an increase in the neural firing rate. It is via this movement of endolymph within the semicircular canals that the vestibule senses rotational acceleration.

Detection of linear acceleration is felt to be accomplished by the otolithic organs, namely, the maculae of the utricle and saccule. Actually the utricle is felt to play the primary role in this function. The role of the saccule has not yet been well described. The otoconia embedded in the gelatinous matrix of the maculae not only give information relative to gravitational field but also, because of inertia and momentum, sense linear acceleration.

The combination of the shape of the utricular macula and the organization of its sensory neuroepithelium allows this organ to sense changes in linear acceleration in any direction. The physical mass of the otoconia is loosely attached to the sensory neuroepithelium via the gelatinous matrix of the macula. At rest this mass is acted upon by gravity, and this effect causes a deflection of the sensory hair cells of the neuroepithelium, allowing us to sense head position relative to gravity. Once movement is initiated in a particular direction, inertia acts on the otoconial mass causing movement of the otoconia relative to the head. This otoconial movement results in a deflection of the neuroepithelial hair cells in the opposite direction from the head's movement. This acceleration (change in velocity over time equals acceleration) is then sensed, and signals are sent to the central nervous system in the form of increased firing rate for some utricular hair cells and decreased firing for others.

This selective stimulation and inhibition of neural firing gives information regarding the direction of movement. Once a steady velocity is reached the otoconia achieve the same velocity as the head, and the firing rate assumes the resting level. If the velocity is changed in the current direction of travel, or the direction of travel is changed, then the otoconia once again move relative to the sensory neuroepithelium. This movement provides new information in the form of hair cell deflection and altered neural firing, which occur as a function of the momentum carried by the otoconia in the original direction of travel.

Processing the complex stream of information provided by the semicircular canals and utricle is accomplished via the vestibular nuclei, cerebellum, and higher centers of the central nervous system. In addition to the information provided by the vestibular system, the central nervous system must also integrate information from visual input and proprioceptive stimuli. It is not yet understood how this integration takes place, nor have the location and roles of all the involved components in the central nervous system been determined. While the lack of a complete understanding of how central integration takes place can frustrate the physician in difficult cases, one can use what is known about symptomatology and vestibular physiology to diagnose the vast majority of patients who present complaining of dizziness.

SUMMARY

In the peripheral vestibular system it is seen that form follows function. It is the orientation of the semicircular canals and the organization of the sensory neuroepithelium within the endolymphatic spaces that allows detection of rotational acceleration. Physicians can take advantage of this relationship in the form of caloric testing to detect signs of vestibular dysfunction. Detection of linear acceleration is accomplished by the utricular macula. Direct testing of this part of the vestibular end organ is not readily accomplished.

Challenges still lie ahead in the understanding of how the central nervous system integrates the multiplicity of sensory inputs related to preserving equilibrium. In spite of the shortcomings in this understanding, physicians can diagnose and treat the majority of patients with balance disorders.

SUGGESTED READING

1. Wolfson (ed). *The vestibular system and its diseases*. Philadelphia: University of Pennsylvania Press, 1966;19–68.
2. Physiology of the vestibular system. In: Cummings C, ed. *Otolaryngology—head and neck surgery*. St. Louis: C.V. Mosby Co, 1986;2679–2721.
3. Conventional bithermal caloric tests. In: Barber HO, Sharpe JA, eds. *Vestibular disorders*. Chicago: Year Book Medical Publishers, Inc., 1988;61–70.

2

Clinical Evaluation of the Vertiginous Patient

History
Neurotologic Examination
    Otologic Examination—Head and Neck · Fistula Test
Examination of the Eyes—Nystagmus
Neurologic Examination
    Cranial Nerves · Cerebellum · Stance and Gait · Positional
    Testing · Audiometric Studies/Auditory Brainstem Response
    (ABR) · Caloric Test · Electronystagmography · Rotational
    Testing · Dynamic Platform Posturography
Radiographic Examination
Hematologic Evaluation
Suggested Reading

As with most cases in medicine, a good history will often make a diagnosis. Such is the case in the initial evaluation of the vertiginous patient. A thorough history will be aided by a complete neurotologic exam establishing the course of future tests leading to and confirming a diagnosis. This chapter reviews the symptoms, the physical exam, and the various tests available to help determine the etiology or site of the lesion. The goal of this chapter is to establish the fundamentals for determining either the site of the lesion (right or left peripheral vestibular, eighth nerve, or central origin), or a non-neurotologic cause (e.g., cardiac or endocrine abnormality).

HISTORY

Dizzy patients often present with an array of confusing complaints and need help organizing their thoughts. A significant

11

amount of time and patience on the examiner's part is required. The first and most important point is to have patients explain in their own words their subjective complaint: "What do you mean you're dizzy?" or "What is that sensation like?"

In general, the patient's symptoms can be placed into the following categories:

Vertigo. A subjective or objective sense of movement often rotatory in nature; usually related to a peripheral labyrinthine cause.

Unsteadiness. Loss of equilibrium often described as "almost falling" or "my balance is off"; the etiology may be abnormalities in the cerebrum, cerebellum, pyramidal track, posterior column, or peripheral system.

Light-headedness. A feeling often related to quick positional changes; usually a vascular etiology.

Dizziness. A disturbed sense of relationship to space in which the etiology may be vestibular, cerebellar, visual, hematologic, or gastrointestinal.

In addition to the patient's characteristic symptom, the initial episode should be described in detail. Other major issues to explore are the following: start of symptoms, activities being performed, length and whether continuous or intermittent, associated symptoms such as nausea or vomiting, frequency at which attacks occur, what brings on symptoms (e.g., change in position) symptoms occurring after the attack, or whether symptoms lessened or resolved completely.

The following information should also be investigated:

1. Associated otologic complaints such as hearing loss—progressive vs. fluctuating, tinnitus, aural fullness, otalgia, otorrhea, or facial paralysis.
2. Previous otologic or nonotologic surgery, head trauma, and noise exposure.
3. Medication history and use of ototoxic and/or vestibular toxic medication.
4. Complete medical history to evaluate the possibility of diabetes, hypothyroidism or hyperthyroidism, cardiovascular disease, eye diseases such as cataracts, and a history of infectious diseases such as measles, mumps, syphilis, etc.

5. Family history to explain possibility of otosclerosis, neurofibromatosis, etc.
6. Central nervous system symptoms such as loss of consciousness, seizure activity, confusion, memory loss, peripheral weakness, numbness, dysphagia, and double, blurred, or loss of vision.

NEUROTOLOGIC EXAMINATION

The neurotologic exam incorporates the head and neck exam and many aspects of the neurologic exam. The following discussion serves as a foundation in the development of the diagnosis. The accompanying worksheet (Table 1) is used to combine the history and physical exam, and to summarize various results.

TABLE 1. *Worksheet for initial evaluation of the vertiginous patient*

Name _____ SEX _____ AGE _____

HISTORY
Chief complaint:
Description:
Onset:
Frequency:
Nausea and vomiting:

HEARING LOSS   R   L
Duration
Progressive
Fluctuating
Tinnitus
Fullness
Better ear

PAST MEDICAL HISTORY

MEDICATIONS
Allergy—medicine sensitivities
Family history

TABLE 1. *Continued*

NEUROTOLOGIC EXAM

BP sitting _____   standing _____

Right ear:

AC>BC   512 Hz   BC>AC
SRT—
Weber   L   Midline   R

Left ear:

AC>BC   512 Hz   BC>AC
SRT—

Nose   Nasopharynx
Oral cavity   Oropharynx
Hypopharynx   Larynx
Neck (bruit)
Heart

Fistula test:
Nystagmus:
Cranial nerves:
Cerebellar function:
Stance and gait:
Positional testing:

SPECIAL TESTING

Audiometric studies/ABR:
Caloric exam:
Electronystagmography:
Rotational testing:
Platform testing:
Radiographic examination
    CT with contrast:
    MRI with gadolinium:
CBC—Blood glucose—5HGTT
Thyroid—triglycerides
Autoimmune
    Sed. rate
    ANA
    RA factor
    LE prep.
    Lymphocyte transformation test
    FTA—ABS

Most often, the examination is performed when the patient is asymptomatic; it is worthwhile to make attempts to examine the patient during or shortly after an attack. Usually, abnormal findings are present only during a vertiginous spell. However, it is important to document the presence or absence of the physical findings discussed below.

Initially, the office nurse should record the patient's pulse and blood pressure sitting and standing, and the general appearance of the patient should be noted.

Otologic Examination—Head and Neck

The auricle and canals are examined to evaluate the possibilities of cerumen impaction, exostoses, osteomas, neoplasms, or malformations. These various lesions will often lead to canal obstruction, which results in hearing loss and often a sense of dizziness or imbalance.

The tympanic membrane is inspected. If any abnormalities are detected using the otoscope, a careful microscopic exam should be performed. In general, patients with vestibular disorders have normal tympanic membranes. The tympanic membranes should be examined for possible serous otitis media, perforations (either traumatic or chronic), evidence of cholesteatoma, hemotympanum suggestive of temporal bone trauma, or painful vesicular eruptions— not only of the tympanic membrane but of the canal and auricle [suggestive of herpes zoster oticus (Ramsay Hunt syndrome)]. The tympanic membrane perforation associated with cholesteatoma can often lead to a fistula formation of the cochlear or vestibular apparatus. Traumatic perforations can be associated with ossicular discontinuity and perilymphatic fistula.

The remainder of the head and neck exam is completed. Often examination of the cranial nerves is incorporated into this portion of the examination and will be discussed later in this chapter.

An estimated speech reception threshold (SRT) is obtained by asking the patient to repeat spondee words (phonetically balanced words such as baseball, cowboy, hot dog) whispered or spoken to one ear. The level at which the patient consistently (greater than 50%) responds correctly is estimated in decibels (dB). A rough esti-

mation of discrimination may also be made. Masking of the contralateral ear may be achieved by the use of a Barony noise box.

Tuning fork testing is performed in all cases and assesses whether
a hearing loss is either conductive or sensorineural. The most common tuning fork used is at 512 Hz. The estimated SRTs, discrimination abilities, and tuning fork tests will serve to confirm the otologic
and audiologic findings.

The Rinne test is performed by placing the vibrating tuning fork
firmly against the mastoid process (bone conduction) and then just
outside the external auditory canal (air conduction). Bone conduction greater than air conduction (negative Rinne) suggests a conductive hearing loss of at least 25 dB. Air conduction greater than bone
conduction (positive Rinne) signifies possible normal hearing, sensorineural hearing loss, or conductive loss smaller than 25 dB.

The Weber test is performed by placing the vibrating tuning fork
on a solid midline surface (forehead, glabella, vertex, or central in-
cisors). The patient determines where the sound is best perceived—
right, left, or midline. The sound will lateralize to the ear with a
conductive hearing loss, the ear with the greater conductive hearing
loss, or away from a sensorineural hearing loss. Therefore in a unilateral hearing loss, sound lateralizing to the better ear suggests a
contralateral sensorineural hearing loss, whereas sound lateralizing
best to the worse ear is characteristic of a conductive hearing loss.

Fistula Test

The fistula test is often employed as a routine part of the neurotologic exam. A positive fistula test is signified by a brief episode of
nystagmus and/or suggestive complaints of motion. In the presence
of chronic otitis media and tympanic membrane perforations, especially in the presence of cholesteatoma, a positive fistula test is in-
dicative of a communication between the middle ear and inner ear
spaces.With an intact tympanic membrane, a positive fistula test
(Hennebert's sign) signifies the presence of adhesions within the inner ear or bony erosion of the otic capsule associated with congenital syphilis, a perilymphatic fistula, or Meniere's disease.

The method of performing a fistula test is performed in several ways. The easiest way is having the patient look straight ahead and applying pressure to the tragus, causing occlusion of the ear canal and creating positive pressure, with subsequent relief. Another method is the use of an olive tip attached to a Politzer's bag. The olive tip is placed in the external auditory canal. Positive and negative pressure are applied, and the patient's eyes are observed with Frenzel's glasses in place. Frenzel's lenses use 20 diopter lenses with accompanied illumination so that the patient is unable to fixate visually and the eyes are under magnification.

Characteristically, a positive fistula test response is greater with positive pressure than with negative pressure. Vertigo is produced when movement of the soft tissue bridging the fistula, such as cholesteatoma, displaces endolymphatic fluid with resultant cupular deviation, as shown in Fig. 1. With an intact tympanic membrane, there is either perilymph or endolymph movement by a resultant bony or perilymph fistula or adhesions in the vestibule between the saccule and stapes footplate, as shown in Fig. 2.

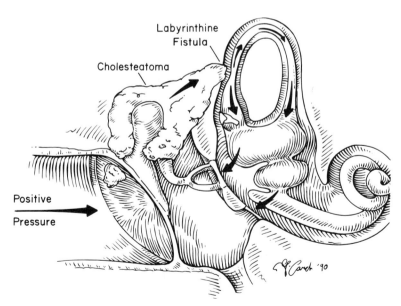

FIG. 1. Cholesteatoma causing labyrinthine fistula.

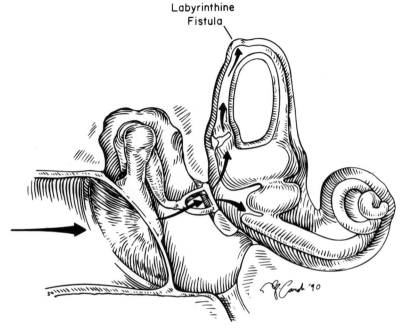

FIG. 2. Endolymphatic movement in bony fistula. Tympanic membrane intact.

EXAMINATION OF THE EYES—NYSTAGMUS

Examination of the eyes may give many important clues to the etiology of vertigo. An arcus senilis is suggestive of vascular insufficiency. An evaluation is made of the visual fields and a fundoscopic examination is performed. Papilledema may be suggestive of a cerebellopontine angle tumor or central disorder causing an increase in intracranial pressure. The extraocular muscles are assessed.

Careful examination should be performed for spontaneous nystagmus. Nystagmus is described by the direction of the fast component, and its presence or absence should be documented. Traditionally, horizontal symptoms nystagmus is characteristic of a peripheral lesion or paresis. Peripheral nystagmus can also be suppressed by visual fixation. To eliminate this visual fixation, Frenzel's glasses are applied.

Rotatory nystagmus is frequently seen with lesions in the vestibular nuclei at the floor of the fourth ventricle. Vertical nystagmus is suggestive of a brainstem lesion. Congenital nystagmus is horizontal and continuous in nature, and the patient generally has no impairment of visual acuity.

Testing of the vestibular ocular reflex can be performed by asking the patient to read from a book while moving the head from side to side. Patients should not have difficulty reading clearly despite this head movement. Intact bilateral vestibular organs should maintain a steady gaze despite head movement. If both vestibular end organs are damaged, the vestibular ocular reflex is lost, and the patient will suffer from oscillopsia—a condition in which objects seem to move back and forth, or the horizon will seem to bounce with each step as they walk.

NEUROLOGIC EXAMINATION

Cranial Nerves

The cranial nerve exam is incorporated into the remainder of the overall head and neck examination. If so indicated, the first cranial nerve is tested using nonirritant odors such as coffee, clove, or tobacco. It is important to remember that mucosal irritants such as alcohol, ammonia, and other chemical substances stimulate sensation by way of the fifth cranial nerve. The second cranial nerve exam includes confrontation testing and the ophthalmoscopic examination. These two provide a check for visual field defects, and the fundus is examined for papilledema. The third, fourth, and sixth cranial nerves are examined by testing the pupillary light reflex , extraocular movements, and checking for ptosis.

The fifth cranial nerve is examined by testing the corneal reflex, proper function of the muscles of mastication, and facial sensation by the use of light touch and pin prick. The seventh cranial nerve is closely inspected for resting symmetry and facial movement. Subtle findings of facial paralysis may be evidenced by a difference in the width of the orbital fissures or flattening of the nasal labial fold. The eighth cranial nerve can be tested by the previously mentioned tuning fork and hearing acuity tests. In addition, vestibular function can be evaluated by caloric examination (to be discussed later). The ninth cranial nerve is evaluated by soft palate function and the gag reflex. The tenth cranial nerve is evaluated during indirect laryngoscopy. The eleventh cranial nerve assesses the function of the trapezius and sternocleidomastoid muscle. Finally, the twelfth cranial nerve is examined for deviation of the tongue, loss of tone, or atrophy.

Cerebellum

Cerebellar function is assessed by several tests with the patient sitting. For example, the finger-to-nose-to-finger test is used to assess possible dysmetria. The patient touches his/her nose and then the examiner's finger. The examiner moves his/her finger in a random fashion. Failure of the patient to hit the nose and the examiner's finger in a consistent manner indicates cerebellar dysfunction. Dysdiadochokinesia is determined by asking the patient to pat the thighs with both hands alternating between the palmer and dorsal surfaces. Rebound is noted by asking the patient to move a limb against resistance and then suddenly removing the resistance. These three tests, along with many others, will assess for cerebellar hemisphere dysfunction. Midline cerebellar disease disrupts the balance and causes gross ataxia, resulting in truncal ataxia or a wide-based gait.

Stance and Gait

The Romberg test is used to assess the spinocerebellar pathways. In this examination, the patient is asked to stand with feet together, arms to the side and eyes closed. The test may be sharpened by asking the subject to extend the arms and stand with the feet in a tandem position. The patient must be able to stand steadily with the eyes opened before a comparison with the eyes closed can be made. The ability to stand with eyes closed depends upon the integrity of the proprioceptive system and functioning spinocerebellar pathway. The test is positive if the patient sways markedly (usually toward the side of the lesion) with the eyes closed. A positive Romberg test usually indicates a posterior column disorder. Patients with a cerebellar disorder have difficulty standing with the eyes opened.

Gait testing is performed by having the patient walk a short distance in a straight line with the eyes opened and then closed. Patients with uncompensated vestibular lesions will deviate toward the side of the lesion.

Positional Testing

Positional testing is a series of maneuvers that attempt to elicit vertigo and nystagmus. Frenzel's glasses are placed on the patient, who is in a sitting position. The head is turned quickly to the right and to the left as far as it will go. If vertigo or nystagmus is elicited, a proprioceptive disorder of the neck is suspected. This may be seen after a whiplash injury. In addition, transitory vascular compromise via the carotid or vertebral arteries may be induced with this maneuver.

Hallpike positional testing is illustrated in Fig. 3. The patient sits on an exmination table in a manner so that when lying down the head will be hanging off the edge. The examiner supports the patient's head throughout the test. With the patient sitting, the initial maneuver is for the patient to lie straight back with the head hanging. Approximately 60 seconds later the patient is brought back to the original sitting position. The patient is instructed to look straight ahead at all times and to keep the eyes open. The next maneuver is to have the patient lie straight back, but this time with the head rotated all the way over to the right. Again, 60 seconds later the patient is brought to the upright position. The maneuver is repeated so that the head is in the left hanging position. In each position the examiner observes the patient for nystagmus.

Several responses can be obtained from this kind of testing. First, direction-fixed positional nystagmus is directed to one side only throughout all position changes. The nystagmus only lasts for a few moments, is fatiguable, and is suggestive of a vestibular end organ disorder.

Direction-changing positional nystagmus takes three different forms. The first type consists of a rotatory nystagmus that begins several seconds upon assuming the head-hanging position and is directed toward the lowermost ear. Thus, with a right head-hanging

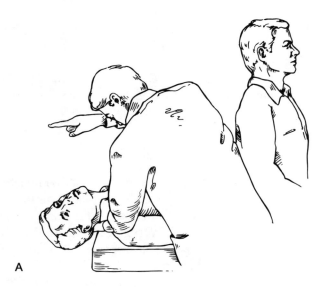

A

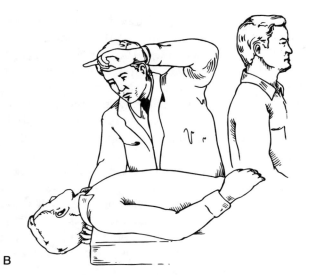

B

FIG. 3. Hallpike positional testing.

position the nystagmus will be in a counterclockwise fashion. With a left head-hanging position the nystagmus will be in a clockwise fashion. Upon sitting upright the rotatory nystagmus reverses direction for a few seconds and then ceases. Subjectively the patient also senses vertigo. These findings are consistent with benign paroxysmal positional vertigo. This condition has been described histopathologically as a result of loose otoconia that have deposited upon the cupula of the posterior semicircular canal (cupulolithiasis).

The second type of direction-changing nystagmus is characteristic of changes in direction with different head-hanging positions. For example, with the right ear down, left beating nystagmus may be visible. The nystagmus changes to right beating in left head-hanging positions. Direction-changing nystagmus of this type is seen with unilateral or bilateral vestibular end organ disorders, but it may occasionally indicate central vestibular dysfunction.

The third form of direction-changing nystagmus is one that changes direction randomly during a single position. This type of response is most suggestive of a central vestibular disorder involving the brainstem.

Audiometric Studies/Auditory Brainstem Response (ABR)

Audiologic studies are a routine integral part of the initial evaluation and are considered an extension of the clinical exam. Pure tone audiometry with air and bone levels with speech reception thresholds are obtained in every patient even if there is no subjective hearing loss. The speech discrimination test is administered to test the understandability of articulated speech.

More specialized audiometric tests may be used to help identify the site of a lesion. Recruitment testing, stapedial reflexes, tone decay, Bekesey audiometry, and the short increment sensitivity index are several of the tests used to determine if the hearing loss is caused by a cochlear or retrocochlear (eighth nerve to auditory cortex) lesion. However, these tests have been replaced for the most part by auditory brainstem response testing and improved imaging techniques, and are mentioned mostly for historical interest.

In some instances, especially when there is asymmetrical sensorineural hearing loss and/or discrimination scores, auditory evoked potentials may be useful components of the diagnostic evaluation.

In the work-up of eighth cranial nerve lesions the auditory brainstem response is particularly useful since it focuses on patterns from the inner ear, eighth nerve, and low brainstem. The procedure is a non-invasive auditory test in which surface electrodes are taped on both ears and the top of the head. Clicks or some suitable stimuli are delivered via earphones and monitored by a signal averager while the patient relaxes or sleeps. The resulting waveforms from both the right and left ears are compared with normal waves and with each other. While both morphology and latency are analyzed, latencies of the waves are the most sensitive indicators. Even small tumors of the cochlear vestibular bundle result in delays between waves I and V in more than 90% of cases. Normal and abnormal wave forms are illustrated in Fig. 4. In this example the upper tracing shows normal waveforms and latencies in the left ear. The lower tracing illustrates

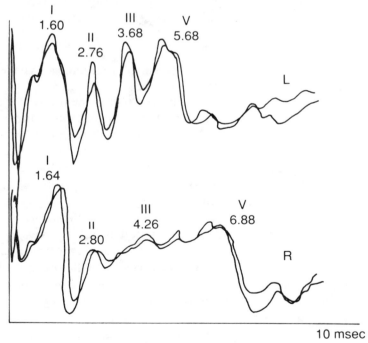

FIG. 4. ABR tracing left ear *(top)* is normal. Right ear *(bottom)* is abnormal.

poor waveform morphology and prolonged latencies consistent with retrocochlear pathology. Because the responses can be obtained, even with the patient under anesthesia, the ABR can also be used to monitor cochlear function during surgery. For example, intraoperative ABR monitoring is used during a vestibular nerve section.

Caloric Test

The vestibular system can be easily and quickly evaluated by the use of the Kobrac minimal caloric test. This is a simple and practical test designed for office use. It is often sufficient for determining labyrinthine function in the routine diagnosis for many vestibular disorders. Frenzel's lenses are placed to prevent ocular fixation. Next, the ear canal and tympanic membrane are examined for possible obstruction and/or perforation. The patient's head is inclined backward at a 60° angle to place the horizontal semicircular canal in a vertical plane, as shown in Fig. 5. Five milliliters of 80°F water are slowly instilled into one of the external auditory canals, as illustrated in

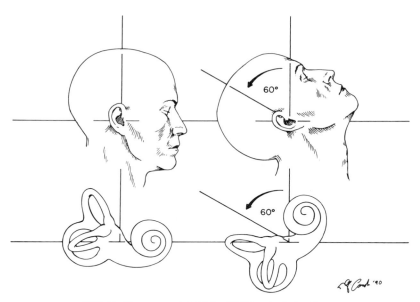

FIG. 5. Proper head tilt for ENG caloric testing.

Fig. 6. This water cools the endolymph and creates a downward current inducing cupular deflection away from the utricle (utriculofugal). This causes nystagmus (fast component) toward the opposite ear. The time of onset and the length of nystagmus are recorded. After 5 to 10 minutes the opposite ear is tested. If no response is obtained with either ear, then 5 cc of ice water is instilled into that ear. If still no further results are obtained, up to 40 cc of ice water is used.

The range of normal responses to thermal calorics is great. Thus it is important to compare the results of both ears in each patient. If there is a reduced response or no response in one ear compared with the other, this indicates a hypoactive or absent vestibular response.

If the sensation produced by the caloric test is exactly the same as the vertigo experienced by the patient, the vertigo is probably of labyrinthine origin. If the patient's dizziness is unlike the sensation produced by the caloric test, the dizziness is probably not due to a labyrinthine lesion, but is of a central origin.

The mnemonic COWS (Cold–Opposite/Warm–Same) is useful in remembering the direction of the nystagmus expected with the use

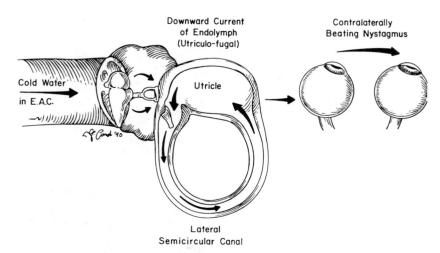

FIG. 6. Cold water causing opposite beating nystagmus.

of either the warm or cold water. For example, if cold water is instilled into the left ear, then right beating nystagmus should occur.

Electronystagmography

Electronystagmography (ENG), which includes caloric testing, is one of the most vital tests for evaluating the vertiginous patient. It is helpful in determining central versus peripheral etiology and in addition, in localizing the dysfunctioning ear. It also serves as a permanent record on the patient's chart of the dysfunctioning ear.

ENG requires approximately 45 to 90 minutes for completion of the test battery. An electrode is placed lateral to each eye with a ground electrode placed on the forehead (Fig. 7). Because of the voltage differences between the cornea and the retina, eye movements can be graphed on a strip chart recording. The equipment permits recording with the patient's eyes closed, thereby eliminating unwanted visual suppression of the diagnostic eye movements. The test battery consists of seven basic procedures.

1. *Saccade test (calibration).*   Calibration of the equipment is accomplished by having the patient look back and forth between two calibration points placed 20° apart. The recorder is adjusted until the pen deflects 20 mm for 20° of eye movement.
2. *Gaze nystagmus tests.*   The patient visually fixates on points, usually lights or dots at 20° and at 30° to the right and to the left.
3. *Sinusoidal eye tracking test.*   The patient visually follows a point moving back and forth along a slow pendular path.
4. *Optokinetic test (OPK).*   The patient observes a pattern of vertical stripes moving horizontally across the visual field. The test is conducted at two to three different speeds, with the stripes moving right to left and left to right.
5. *Positional tests.*   The patient is monitored while in a variety of head and body positions. Eye movements are recorded with eyes open and with eyes closed for 30 seconds in each position. The patient is first observed when seated erect with the head straight and eyes closed. Nystagmus present in this position is called "spontaneous nystagmus," as there are no nystagmus-inducing stimuli. Nystagmus present in other positions is called "positional nystagmus." Common positions tested are:

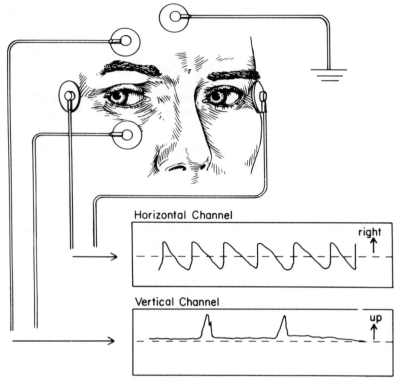

FIG. 7. ENG electrode placement and tracing.

    a. Supine with head straight, with head right and with head left.
    b. Supine with the whole body right and the whole body left.
    c. Sitting with the head left, with head right, with head hanging down and with head extended backwards.

6. *Hallpike positional test.* The patient is rapidly moved from a sitting to a supine head-hanging position and after approximately 30 seconds, is returned to the sitting position. The maneuver is repeated from a sitting to a right head-hanging position and then left head-hanging position.

7. *Bithermal caloric test.* With the patient's head inclined backward 60° (if patient is sitting) and with eyes closed, each ear is irrigated separately with cool and warm water or air. Approxi-

mately 30 seconds after the response to the caloric stimulation begins, the patient is asked to fixate on a stationary spot or point for about 10 seconds and then close his/her eyes again. When an ear is irrigated with the cool stimulus, the fast phase of the nystagmus should beat in the opposite direction of the ear that is irrigated. With the warm stimulus, the fast phase should beat toward the irrigated ear. Observations of the nystagmus resulting from the four stimulations are made in terms of its direction, duration, frequency, and speed of the slow component.

The various tests, abnormal findings, reliability, and localizing values for each are shown in Table 2.

Rotational Testing

Since the early 1970s, there has been a great deal of interest in the development and improvement of rotational techniques for testing. Since rotational acceleration is the physiologic stimulus to the semicircular canals during natural movements of the head, it has been used for vestibular testing since the early 1900s. Recent advancements in hydraulic systems, ENG electrodes that accurately document eye position relative to the chair position, and, most importantly, computer analysis of these eye positions and velocity done over multiple cycles of sinusoidal stimulation have brought rotatory chair testing out of the laboratory and into the clinical spectrum.

The current value of rotational testing is found in three areas: first, the discovery of a vestibular abnormality unrecognized by conventional vestibular testing; secondly, providing additional information before relegating the patient to a diagnosis of psychogenic vertigo; finally, monitoring the progression of the central compensatory mechanism.

However, because of the cost and controversies still centering around the optimal test frequencies and nature of the stimulus, this test is not widely used or considered part of the routine evaluation. Results of ongoing studies are encouraging and support the concept that computer analysis of rotatory test data will yield more valuable information regarding central and peripheral vestibular function in the future.

TABLE 2. *Summary of ENG abnormalities*

Test and abnormality	Location of lesion
Saccade test	
1. Multiple-step saccades	Always CNS (cerebellar system)
2. Hypermetric saccades	Always CNS (cerebellar system)
3. Flutter	Always CNS (brainstem)
4. Internuclear opthalmoplegia	Always CNS (medial longitudinal fasciculus)
5. Slowing	Always CNS
Gaze test	
1. Spontaneous nystagmus, suppressed by visual fixation	Usually peripheral vestibular system (ear opposite direction on nystagmus
2. Spontaneous nystagmus, not suppressed by visual fixation	Always CNS
3. Gaze-paretic nystagmus	
a. Unilateral	Always CNS
b. Bilateral	Always CNS
4. Brun's nystagmus	Usually brainstem compression on side of gaze nystagmus)
5. Congenital nystagmus	Always CNS (benign)
6. Square wave jerks	Always CNS (cerebellar system)
7. Periodic alternating nystagmus	Always CNS
8. Rebound nystagmus	Always CNS (cerebellar system)
9. Downbeating nystagmus	Always CNS (cerebellum or lower brainstem)
10. Upbeating nystagmus	Always CNS (cerebellum or medulla
Tracking test	
1. Saccadic tracking	Always CNS
Optokinetic test	
1. Weak response	
a. Unilateral	Always CNS
b. Bilateral	Always CNS
2. Inversion	(Seen only in patients with congenital nystagmus)
Positional test	
1. Positional nystagmus, suppressed by visual fixation	
a. Direction-fixed	Peripheral vestibular system (either ear) or CNS
b. Direction-changing in different head positions	Peripheral vestibular system (either ear) or CNS
c. Direction-changing in single head position	Always CNS
2. Positional nystagmus, not suppressed by visual fixation	Always CNS
Hallpike maneuver	
1. Benign paroxysmal positional nystagmus	
a. Unilateral	Usually peripheral vestibular system (undermost ear)
b. Bilateral	Usually peripheral vestibular system (both ears)
2. Any other nystagmus	Usually CNS
Caloric test	
1. Unilateral weakness	Always peripheral vestibular system (weak ear)
2. Directional preponderance	Peripheral vestibular system (either ear) or CNS
3. Bilateral weakness	Usually peripheral vestibular system (both ears)
4. Failure of fixation suppression	Always CNS
5. Caloric inversion	Always CNS
6. Caloric perversion	Always CNS

Dynamic Platform Posturography

Platform testing relies on the hypothesis that three sensory inputs are responsible for balance; labyrinthine, proprioception, and vision. Computerized platform testing is now commercially available with the use of the Equitest manufactured by Neurocom International, Inc.

The patient stands with each foot on a special sensor plate. Sensors from each corner detect body sway and feed the data to a computer for analysis. The footplate and the wall of the booth in which the subject optically fixates can be moved and are sway references. Six different conditions are investigated:

1. Eyes open, platform stable, visual field stable
2. Eyes shut, platform stable (Romberg test)
3. Eyes open, platform stable, visual field swayed
4. Eyes open, platform swayed, visual field stable
5. Eyes shut, platform stable
6. Eyes open, platform swayed, visual field swayed

These various tests allow for evaluation of one, two, or all three mechanisms responsible for balance.

It has been suggested that this test can distinguish between three types of vestibular function:

1. Bilaterally or unilaterally reduced labyrinthine function
2. Fluctuations in vestibular function, such as those accompanying endolymphatic hydrops or perilymph fistula
3. Distortion of vestibular reflex function of the benign paroxysmal positional nystagmus type

At this time, platform testing is supplemental and is not widely used because of the expense of the computerized system that is now commercially available. However, its use does appear to be more accepted and widespread. The exam seems most useful in those patients with a borderline normal or normal clinical testing and rotary testing results. Both the rotatory chair and the platform test have become fairly routine in very specialized vestibular disorder clinics throughout the country.

RADIOGRAPHIC EXAMINATION

Magnetic resonance imaging (MRI) with gadolinium injection is now the primary mode in the investigation of the cerebellopontine angle, posterior fossa, and cranial vertebral abnormalities. The contents of these areas are better demonstrated by MRI than by computed tomography (CT). The CT scan with or without contrast is still imperative when the bony structures of the temporal bone need to be evaluated.

MRI with gadolinium injection is obtained on all patients where there is a high index of suspicion for cerebellopontine angle tumors. This would include patients who have abnormal ABR testing, asymmetrical sensorineural hearing loss, and asymmetrical discrimination scores. If the patient cannot submit to the MRI examination, then CT with contrast is still acceptable for the evaluation of the cerebellopontine angle area, but it fails to pick up the smaller tumors that can be seen on MRI.

HEMATOLOGIC EVALUATION

The following tests serve as a general guideline to the hematologic evaluation. CBC, blood glucose, and 5-hour glucose tolerance test, thyroid function, triglycerides, cholesterol, and FTA–ABS can be routinely ordered during the initial evaluation or when the vertiginous symptoms are not responsive to standard treatment. Depending upon the clinical history, an autoimmune evaluation may incorporate the following tests: Complete Blood Count, Erythrocyte Sedimentation Rate; Fluorescent Treponemal Antibody-Absorption Test, Antinuclear Antibodies, Rheumatoid Factor, Raji cell assay, Ciq Binding Assay, CH_{50} and Western Blot Assay to inner ear antigens. The lymphocyte transformation test is a highly specialized test and is only performed at select centers in the United States. This is still thought to be an experimental test by many. Another test available only in research centers is the Western blot immunoprecipitation test for anticochlear antibodies. This test can identify the presence of antibodies directed against the cochlea or with cross reactivity to cochlear antigens.

SUGGESTED READING

1. Cummings C. *Otolaryngology—head and neck surgery*. St. Louis: CV Mosby Co, 1986.
2. Alberti P, Reuben R. *Otologic Medicine and Surgery*. New York: Churchill Livingstone Co, 1988.
3. Barrow H. *Guide to neurological assessment*. Philadelphia: JB Lippincott Co, 1980.
4. DeJong R. *The neurologic examination*. Philadelphia: Harper and Row Co, 1979.
5. Glasscock M, Jackson C, Josey F. *The ABR handbook*. New York: Thieme, 1987.
6. Shambaugh G, Glasscock M. *Surgery of the Ear*. Philadelphia: WB Saunders Co, 1980.
7. Barber HO, Stockwell CW. *Manual of electronystagmography*. St Louis: CV Mosby, 1980.
8. Hart CW. *Manual of electronystagmography*. Washington: American Academy of Otolaryngology—Head and Neck Surgery Foundation Inc., 1987.
9. Black FO. Vestibulospinal function assessment by moving platform posturography. *Am J Otol,* 1985;7 (Supp):39.

3

Peripheral Vestibular Disorders

Symptoms of disequilibrium can be an enigma to both the patient and physician. The symptoms, the manner in which they occur, their duration, and many other factors must be assessed to differentiate from among the numerous potential peripheral and central causes of dizziness, vertigo, and imbalance. An understanding of the fundamentals of normal vestibular anatomy and physiology is crucial to one's ability to correlate the symptoms and findings and arrive at a diagnosis. Chapters 1 and 2 strive to provide this essential background and are recommended reading as a prelude to this chapter.

This chapter discusses the most common peripheral disorders that present with vertigo. The clinical manifestations and pathophysiology of Meniere's disease, labyrinthitis, vestibular neuronitis, benign paroxysmal positional vertigo (BPPV), perilymphatic fistula, and autoimmune vestibulopathy are discussed. The general diagnostic characteristics of each entity are reviewed to help facilitate their recognition.

35

MENIERE'S DISEASE

In 1861, contrary to current thinking, Prosper Meniere ascribed the symptom complex that bears his name to the inner ear rather than the central nervous system. In his original paper he described these paroxysms of vertigo accompanied by tinnitus and hearing loss as a seizure of the inner ear. New insight into the pathologic process of Meniere's disease was provided by Hallpike and Cairns in 1938 when they described the finding of endolymphatic hydrops as a consistent pathological finding in patients with the disease. Since that time considerable efforts have been made by numerous investigators in the attempt to uncover the underlying etiologic factor(s) that cause this disease. Continued work is needed and indeed is under way; the reader is encouraged to keep abreast of the latest developments.

In general, Meniere's disease has its onset in the third or fourth decade of life and affects the sexes equally. It most commonly affects only one ear, but published rates of bilateral involvement range between 20% and 40%. Typically the patient with Meniere's disease has a triad of symptoms in a characteristic classical pattern of episodic true vertigo (vertigo being defined as the sensation of spinning), preceded by a building pressure sensation in one ear, accompanied by increasing tinnitus and diminishing hearing. At the time of the vertiginous spell, nausea and vomiting are often present. This severe disequilibrium (vertigo) will persist anywhere from approximately 30 minutes to 24 hours. Gradually the severe symptoms will abate and the patient is generally ambulatory within 72 hours. Some sensation of instability will persist for days or weeks, and then normal balance will return. During this recuperation time, hearing gradually returns. It may return to the preattack baseline or there may be residual permanent sensorineural hearing loss, most commonly in the lower frequencies. Tinnitus will also usually diminish as the hearing returns. As the disease progresses, hearing fails to return after the attacks, and after many years the symptoms of vertigo may gradually diminish in frequency and severity.

Variations from this idealized history are common, but the characteristics most critical to the diagnosis are: episodic true vertigo, fluctuating hearing loss (usually low-frequency), tinnitus in the affected ear (often fluctuating or even crescendo prior to attacks), and the sensation of aural pressure in the involved ear. An auxiliary symptom, which can be helpful at times, is recruitment in the involved ear.

Useful diagnostic tests include the audiogram and electronystagmography (ENG). Typically the audiogram displays a unilateral sensorineural hearing loss involving the lower frequencies of the involved ear. Fluctuation in discrimination scores is often seen, with a long-term trend toward poor scores. ENG may or may not demonstrate a unilateral vestibular weakness on caloric testing, again involving the ear symptomatic for pressure, hearing loss, and tinnitus. Electrocochleography is useful in cases that are unclear. The finding of enlarged summating potentials in the suspected ear is diagnostic of endolymphatic hydrops.

A BERA must be done in those cases with findings of retrocochlear pathology on routine audiometry to screen for cochlear nerve or brainstem pathology. Such pathology could include an acoustic neuroma or multiple sclerosis. If the BERA is found to be positive, then magnetic resonance imaging (MRI) scanning with the use of intravenous gadolinium should be done to assess for the CNS pathology or eighth nerve schwannoma.

Variations on the classic history exist, which can be categorized as ''cochlear Meniere's'' and ''vestibular Meniere's.'' Cochlear Meniere's is characterized by the symptoms of fluctuating hearing loss, tinnitus, and aural pressure involving one ear. Essentially all of the symptoms of Meniere's disease are present except the vertigo and accompanying nausea and vomiting. In vestibular Meniere's the symptoms of episodic vertigo and aural fullness are reported without hearing loss or fluctuation in hearing. The presence of tinnitus is variable.

Current theory regarding the pathophysiologic mechanism of Meniere's disease identifies the presence of endolymphatic hydrops as a consistent pathologic finding in patients with the disease. It is, however, still unclear whether endolymphatic hydrops itself is the cause of the symptoms characteristic of Meniere's disease or whether it is a pathologic change seen in the disease. The anatomic changes of endolymphatic hydrops are felt to be related to abnormalities in endolymphatic homeostasis. Controversy continues on whether it is overproduction or defective reabsorption of endolymph that causes the hydrops.

Using the concept of endolymphatic hydrops as the pathologic process that results in the symptoms allows a theoretic correlation between anatomic events and symptoms. One can envision the endolymphatic pressure building, causing the feeling of aural fullness. With this building pressure, movement of the basement membrane by auditory stimulation becomes dampened, causing the loss in hearing. Tinnitus would become louder as hearing is affected. Then when the endolymphatic pressure reaches a critical level, a rupture in Reissner's membrane occurs. This rupture allows mixing of the chemically different endolymph and perilymph, causing a loss of membrane potential at the neuroepithelium. The loss of membrane potential thus causes a cessation of neural activity on the affected side. Such acute hypofunctioning of the vestibule causes the severe vertigo and associated vegetative symptoms. The nystagmus seen in an acute attack is paralytic in nature. This scenario is very appealing, but scientific investigation suggests that the situation is more complex. Recent evidence suggests that endolymphatic hydrops may not be responsible for the symptoms and is, instead, a consequence of the underlying pathologic condition that is causing the symptoms. Many potential etiologies have been put forward as causes of Meniere's disease; none have yet been definitively proved.

LABYRINTHITIS

Viral labyrinthitis is the most common form of labyrinthitis seen in clinical practice. Its onset is often preceded by the presence of a viral infection of the upper respiratory or gastrointestinal tracts. The associated viral infection may be coincident with the labyrinthitis or may have preceded it by as much as 2 weeks. The initial symptoms are severe true vertigo that is exacerbated by movement of the head. Hearing loss is not usually present, but when present it should alert the physician to consider other diagnoses in the differential (i.e., Meniere's disease, acoustic neuroma, CNS pathology, serous labyrinthitis, or neurosyphilis). If examined early, the patient may manifest an irritative nystagmus from the acute phases of the viral inflammation. Usually the patient is examined after these initial findings have given way to a more paralytic, or hypofunctional, pattern. The symptoms usually abate after a period of 48 to 72 hours and gradual return to normal balance occurs over approximately 6 weeks.

The differential diagnosis should initially include other causes of vertigo, and careful history taking, physical examination, and an audiogram are required. Physical examination should include neurological examination with attention to cranial nerve findings and cerebellar testing. Careful otoscopy is performed to rule out the presence of a potential otologic infectious process as the source of a toxic serous labyrinthitis. Acute otitis media or cholesteatoma can result in a toxic or even suppurative labyrinthitis. Differentiating between toxic and suppurative labyrinthitis can be difficult at times and requires careful vigilance in suspected cases. Fever in the presence of chronic ear disease and labyrinthitis suggests suppuration and meningitis. Fortunately, toxic and suppurative labyrinthitis from infectious causes are uncommon in the antibiotic era. More typically a toxic labyrinthitis is the result of a well-defined event such as surgery or trauma.

VESTIBULAR NEURONITIS

Controversy exists as to whether vestibular neuronitis exists or whether the symptoms represent a form of chronic labyrinthitis. History of a precipitating viral infection may be elicited. However, the differentiating factor is the recurrent nature of the attacks without accompanying symptoms that would suggest another diagnosis. Theoretically, vestibular neuronitis is an indolent viral inflammation affecting the vestibular nerve. The affected patient is prone to episodic exacerbations with vertigo symptoms unaccompanied by aural pressure, hearing loss, or tinnitus. The attacks are similar to recurrent bouts of viral labyrinthitis and have the same clinical course. Establishing the offending ear can be difficult unless the patient can be examined early during an episode, at which time ENG testing may show a unilateral weakness on caloric testing.

BENIGN PAROXYSMAL POSITIONAL VERTIGO

Benign paroxysmal positional vertigo (BPPV) is indeed a distinct clinical entity; however, its pathophysiology remains incompletely understood. Typically, a patient with BPPV will complain of true vertigo, the onset of which is rapidly brought about by assuming sometimes very specific head positions. Most commonly these head positions involve extension of the neck, often with the head turned to one side. The symptoms are often encountered while rolling from side to side in bed. If questioned carefully the patient may be able to volunteer that the vertigo will only last 1 to 2 minutes and will go away if the precipitating position is maintained. Hearing loss, aural fullness, and tinnitus are not seen in this condition. It most commonly occurs spontaneously in the elderly population, and can occur in any age group after even mild head trauma.

Evaluation should include a careful neurotologic examination, the most important part being the history. Audiometry should be done for completeness. A key diagnostic maneuver is the Dix–Hallpike positioning test. This may be done in combination with ENG monitoring. Often all that is necessary is a pair of Frenzel lenses. Using these lenses the clinician can often observe the pathomnemonic rotatory nystagmus beating toward the dependent ear when the offending position is assumed. This finding suggests that the dependent ear is the diseased ear.

This condition is usually self-limited and will commonly resolve spontaneously within 6 to 12 months. Simple exercises can speed recovery; however, occasionally medication is necessary to control symptoms. The classic explanation of the underlying pathophysiology (cupulolithiasis) was described by Schuknecht in 1969. His study of the temporal bones of two patients afflicted with this disorder showed deposition of otoconial material in the cupula of the posterior semicircular canal. Further support of this etiology is the relief of symptoms obtained by sectioning the posterior ampullary nerve in those patients with persistent problems after conservative treatment. There has been some controversy as to whether this pathologic finding is indeed the cause of symptoms in these patients.

If symptoms persist longer than expected, then further investigation such as an MRI scan should be done to assess for unusual causes of positional vertigo such as acoustic neuroma or tumors of the fourth ventricle.

PERILYMPHATIC FISTULA

By definition, perilymphatic fistula is a disruption of the limiting membranes of the labyrinth. Most commonly these fistulas are found to occur through the round and oval windows of the middle ear. (For the purpose of this discussion we will address fistulas of the round and oval windows, having touched upon fistulas relating to cholesteatoma in the section on labyrinthitis.) Classically, a history of head trauma, barotrauma to the ears, penetrating injury to the tympanic membrane, or vigorous straining proceeds the onset of sudden vertigo, hearing loss, and loud tinnitus. The patient will often report a ''pop'' in the ear during the precipitating event. The symptoms will often subside while at rest only to resume with activity. Sneezing, straining, nose blowing, and other such maneuvers can elicit the symptoms after the initial event.

Physical examination, particularly otoscopy, is important. In the cases of head trauma and barotrauma, hemotympanum is often seen as an early finding. In cases of penetrating injury to the ear, a tympanic membrane perforation makes the likelihood of ossicular discontinuity with fistula very high. Audiometric findings usually demonstrate a mixed or sensorineural hearing loss, depending on the mechanism of injury. This loss may be quite severe and usually involves the high frequencies more than the low frequencies. ENG with caloric testing may be normal or show a unilateral weakness in the affected ear. A clinical fistula test is performed by varying barometric pressure in the external auditory canal and by trying to elicit nystagmus, vertigo, or feeling of imbalance. The specificity of this test can be augmented by the use of ENG monitoring or posturography monitoring during the examination. In spite of refinements, this test remains unreliable in detecting all fistulae. The diagnosis remains, essentially, a historical one, and in those patients with a suggestive history and symptoms treatment is indicated. Often the only manner in which the diagnosis is made definitively is at the time of surgical exploration.

AUTOIMMUNE VESTIBULOPATHY

Autoimmune conditions affecting the inner ear are a rare but distinct clinical entity. First described in 1979 by McCabe, they are characterized by a progressive, bilateral sensorineural hearing loss often accompanied by a bilateral loss of vestibular function. Other autoimmune-mediated disease is often present in the afflicted patients; examples include rheumatoid arthritis, psoriasis, ulcerative colitis, Cogan's syndrome (iritis accompanied by vertigo and SNHL*). The history is the most useful diagnostic tool. Support for the diagnosis can be obtained by blood testing for complete blood count, erythrocyte sedimentation rate, rheumatoid factor, and antinuclear antibodies. Western blot precipitation studies to look for anticochlear antibodies can be done in some research centers and may be the future definitive test of choice in these cases.

Little is known about how this condition causes otologic symptoms. As with other autoimmune conditions, it may occur as a direct assault by the immune system in the form of humoral and cellular immunity directed at the inner ear. Another mechanism of injury may be related to the deposition of antibody–antigen complex in capillaries or basement membranes of inner ear structures. Further immunologic studies of temporal bones harvested from deceased patients who had clinical evidence of autoimmune inner ear involvement may shed some light on the underlying process.

SUMMARY

The characteristic features and pathophysiology of the most common peripheral vestibular disorders presenting with vertigo have been discussed. It is hoped that with a basic appreciation of vestibular anatomy and physiology the clinical manifestations of these diseases will be better understood. Information on vestibular dysfunction will change at a rapid pace as more research is directed toward discovering the mechanisms of normal function and disease processes. The clinician must make continuous efforts to keep abreast of the new data to provide the best of care to those patients with disequilibrium and vertigo.

---

*SNHL, sensorineural hearing loss.

SUGGESTED READINGS

1. Rauch SD, Merchant SN, Thedinger BA, Meniere's syndrome and endolymphatic hydrops: double-blind temporal bone study. *Ann Otol Rhinol Laryngol* 1989;98:873.
2. Schuknecht HF. Cupulolithiasis. *Arch Otolaryngol* 1969;90:765.
3. Gacek RR. Transection of the posterior ampullary nerve for relief of benign paroxysmal positional vertigo. *Ann Otol* 1974;83:596.
4. McCabe BF. Autoimmune sensorineural hearing loss. *Ann Otol Rhinol Laryngol* 1979;88:585.

4

Central Disorders That Cause Vertigo

Vascular Disorders
    Vertebro–Basilar Insufficiency (VBI) · Posterior Fossa Migraine
    · Vascular Loop Syndrome · Vaso-occlusive Disease
Multiple Sclerosis (MS)
CNS Neoplasms
Summary
Suggesting Reading

A number of central nervous system disorders can mimic dysfunction of the peripheral vestibular organ. This chapter covers a number of the most common central conditions that manifest as disequilibrium. Their distinguishing clinical features and helpful diagnostic tests are discussed.

VASCULAR DISORDERS

Probably the most common central cause of vertigo is the broad category of vascular disorders, including vertebro–basilar insufficiency, posterior fossa migraine, vascular loop syndrome, and vaso–occlusive disease.

Vertebro–Basilar Insufficiency (VBI)

In the elderly population, this entity may well prove to be a common cause of vertigo. Usually the onset of symptoms is rapid, lasting several minutes, and the vertigo is often accompanied by nausea and vomiting. Other associated symptoms include visual changes (brown-out), drop attacks, weakness, visual field defects or hallucinations, diplopia, and headaches. Diminished blood flow to the posterior cerebral circulation is the direct cause of symptoms. The varied etiologies that can cause this diminished blood flow include atherosclerotic vascular disease in the subclavian, vertebral, and/or basilar arteries. Orthostatic hypotension, mechanical compression, and Stokes-Adams attacks can result in vertebro–basilar insufficiency. A rare cause of VBI is subclavian steal syndrome, in which vestibular symptoms can be brought on by exercise of the upper extremities.

The patient's age, history of symptoms (vertigo and associated symptoms), and any precipitating events should lead one to the diagnosis, after other causes have been ruled out. Angiography is not routinely ordered, but can be useful in establishing a tenuous diagnosis or in the event of anticipated surgical intervention. However, the risks associated with cerebral angiography must be kept in mind before ordering the study.

Posterior Fossa Migraine

Posterior fossa migraine has been recognized as a migraine variant since 1961. The clinical picture is characterized by an aura, which results from ischemia in the distribution of the basilar artery. Visual disturbances commonly occur, since the basilar artery supplies the occipital and posterior temporal lobes of the brain. Symptoms of temporary diplopia, tinnitus, vertigo, dysarthria and, rarely, hearing loss result from dysfunction of cranial nerves three–twelve. Sensorimotor signs of weakness, drop attacks, paresthesia of the extremities or face, and even syncope are described.

This problem can easily be confused with peripheral vestibular disease, since the onset of vertigo is abrupt and may last from 5 to 60 minutes. The headache that typically follows can be mild, and the patient may overlook it as a symptom during the history taking. Trying to elicit the other typical aura symptoms is helpful in establishing the diagnosis since these symptoms cannot be explained by isolated vestibular end organ dysfunction. Other important factors to consider are a previous history of migraine headaches in the patient or family, audiogram results (usually normal), and electronystagmography (ENG) results (usually normal). This is a diagnosis primarily made on the history, since there are no objective tests for migraine disorders.

Vascular Loop Syndrome

Controversy still surrounds the proposed relationship between the presence of vascular loops in the cerebellopontine angle and symptoms of vertigo and sometimes hearing loss. This is a diagnosis reached often after a number of other etiologies have been excluded. The symptoms can mimic Meniere's syndrome in many ways. Physical exertion can bring on symptoms, which are believed to be related to increased cardiac output causing increased pressure on the eighth nerve by the encroaching blood vessel, usually described as the anterior inferior cerebellar artery or one of its branches making a loop into the internal auditory canal. An ectatic basilar artery compressing the eighth nerve root entry zone has also been implicated. Often no hearing loss or vestibular weakness is found on audiometric testing. The presence of a vascular loop can be suggested by MRI but it most convincingly demonstrated with a CT scan using both intravenous contrast and air cisternography at the same time.

Vaso–occlusive Disease

Acute ischemic insults to the brainstem and cerebellum usually result in dramatic symptoms, which often include vertigo, nausea, and vomiting. Differentiating these events from vestibular end organ dysfunction is facilitated by the presence of associated findings of central injury. The lateral medullary syndrome, caused by infarction in the distribution of the anterior inferior cerebellar artery (AICA), is characterized by vertigo and nausea, as well as ataxia, ipsilateral Horner's syndrome, loss of pain and temperature sensation of the ipsilateral face and contralateral body, and ipsilateral palatal, pharyngeal, and laryngeal paralysis.

Cerebellar infarction can initially present as acute labyrinthine disorder, since the early symptoms are severe vertigo, nausea, vomiting, and ataxia. The distinguishing features are the gait and extremity ataxia and gaze paretic nystagmus. If undiagnosed, the cerebellum can swell, causing progressive brainstem dysfunction and eventual death if surgical decompression is not undertaken.

More insidious, and probably more common in the elderly population, is the effect of small lacunar infarcts that by themselves are not necessarily symptomatic. However, when multiple infarcts have occurred in the region of the pons and brainstem, imbalance can be a very common complaint. The lacunar syndrome, found most frequently in patients with hypertension and documented atherosclerotic vascular disease, can manifest in many ways. Dizziness is one of its manifestations. The diagnosis is most readily made on CT scan or MRI of the brain with fine cuts through the posterior fossa.

MULTIPLE SCLEROSIS (MS)

This demyelinating disease of the central nervous system is a capricious entity of as yet unknown etiology. Its hallmark is the finding of multiple signs of disseminated CNS dysfunction, which may occur over time. While vertigo will occur as the initial symptom of MS in only 5% of patients, it is reported by 50% of patients some time during the course of the disease. Another common symptom of MS is visual loss or blurring due to optic nerve demyelination. Visual complaints are the presenting symptoms for 20% of MS patients. While no specific test for MS exists, abnormalities in CSF gamma globulin (elevated) and elevated CSF myelin basic protein are found in 90% of patients. With advances in imaging technology, MRI may become the diagnostic test of choice in the identification of areas of demyelination in the CNS.

CNS NEOPLASMS

For the purposes of this book, schwannomas of the eighth cranial nerve (acoustic neuromas) will be considered as tumors of the central nervous system. While these tumors typically present with unilateral progressive sensorineural hearing loss and tinnitus, they can also cause vertigo and sudden hearing loss and mimic an attack of Meniere's syndrome. Abnormalities in audiometric impedance batteries should alert the physician to the possibility of retrocochlear pathology. Brainstem-evoked response audiometry is an excellent and cost-effective screening tool for acoustic neuromas. However, since the availability of gadolinium as a contrast agent used with MRI, this study has become the gold standard in the diagnosis of these tumors. MRI scanning with gadolinium can accurately diagnose lesions of the internal auditory canal as small as 3 to 4 mm. Symptoms that should heighten a clinician's suspicion for an acoustic neuroma are unilateral or asymmetric SNHL, unilateral tinnitus, asymmetric discrimination scores, and facial numbness or tingling. Meningiomas arising in the cerebellopontine angle can be difficult to distinguish from an acoustic neuroma and must be considered in the differential diagnosis.

Brainstem gliomas or benign astrocytomas can present with symptoms of labyrinthine dysfunction related to involvement of the vestibular nuclei; however, the usual presence of other associated brainstem findings suggests a central process. As with other CNS neoplasms, MRI appears to be the most sensitive means of diagnosis. The typical history is of relentless progression of brainstem dysfunction, eventually affecting the vital cardiorespiratory centers of the medulla, resulting in death. These tumors have a five to ten times higher incidence in children than adults.

SUMMARY

Careful attention to the history and salient features of physical examination will often allow the clinician to differentiate a central from a peripheral etiology. Appropriate testing is also helpful in establishing the correct diagnosis. Fortunately, the majority of central causes of vertigo are amenable to different forms of therapy. Most of these can be treated by the otolaryngologist. However, neurologic consultation may be necessary in the management of central causes of vertigo.

SUGGESTED READING

1. Fischer CM. Vertigo in cerebrovascular disease. *Arch Otolaryngol* 1967;85:529.
2. Bickerstaff ER. Basilar artery migraine. *Lancet* 1961;1:15.
3. Bartleson JD. Transient and persistent neurological manifestations of migraine. *Stroke* 1984;15:383.
4. McCabe BF, Harker LA. Vascular loop as a cause of vertigo. *Ann Otol Rhinol Laryngol* 1983;92:542.

5

Treatment of Vertigo

Medical Management of Vertigo
  Meniere's Disease · Labyrinthitis · Vestibular Neuronitis ·
  Benign Paroxysmal Positional Vertigo · Autoimmune
  Vestibulopathy · Vascular Vertigo
Surgical Management of Vertigo
  Meniere's Disease · Benign Paroxysmal Positional Vertigo ·
  Perilymph Fistula · Vascular Loop Syndrome
Summary
Suggested Reading

Treatment of the vertiginous patient must take into account the etiology and severity of symptoms. This chapter discusses the treatment rationales for the most common causes of vertigo. Both medical and surgical treatment options are covered, along with their indications. The first section addresses medical management of the vertiginous patient, it is followed by a discussion of surgical treatment of vertigo.

MEDICAL MANAGEMENT OF VERTIGO

Meniere's Disease

Meniere's disease is probably the most common cause of vertigo seen by the otolaryngologist. Keeping in mind the theoretic pathophysiology of Meniere's disease, regulation of dietary salt intake combined with the use of diuretics should be the first focus of treatment. The goal of this therapy is to minimize fluid and salt retention, which may have a destabilizing effect in the inner ear. In particular, the restriction of salt intake must be strongly stressed to the patient in order to maximize compliance. Taking the time to explain the pathophysiology in simple terms allows patients to understand the treatment rationale and will improve the likelihood that they will cooperate in their care. Providing patients with easily obtained reference material regarding the salt content of foods will heighten their awareness and ability to avoid offending foods. (See references 22 and 23 for dietary information sources.) In addition to limited salt intake, patients should avoid the use of tobacco and caffeine-containing products.

Adjunctive medications in the form of vestibular suppressants are to be used primarily during the acute episodes of vertigo and should be discouraged as a chronic daily medication, except in rare cases. The first-line vestibular suppressants include antihistamines, phenothiazines, and anticholinergics. Meclizine (Antivert), diphenhydramine (Benadryl), promethazine (Phenergan), scopolamine (Transderm Scop), glycopyrolate (Robinul), and others can be given in oral or suppository forms and are effective in the majority of patients. These medications have a low incidence of serious side effects and are relatively inexpensive.

The next level of vestibular suppressants would be benzodiazepines such as diazepam (Valium), prazepam (Centrax), and alprazolam (Xanax). These agents provide strong vestibular suppression but have a higher likelihood of side effects and potential addiction problems. Usually low doses of benzodiazepines are sufficient to control vertigo that is not well controlled on the first level of medications.

For severe cases of vertigo that are, unresponsive to benzodiazepines, hospitalization and more potent medications may be necessary. These potent vestibular suppressants include droperidol (Inapsine) and diphenidol (Vontrol). Droperidol (Inapsine) is administered intravenously at doses from 0.75 mg to 1.5 mg in adults. The initial dose is usually 0.75 mg and if effective is not repeated unless vertigo returns. If there is no relief within 6 hours after the first dose, then the next dose is increased by 0.25 mg to 0.75 mg, depending on the patient's weight. Hypotension and a sense of anxiety are the most common side effects. An uncommon but highly distressing group of side effects involves the extrapyramidal central nervous system and includes dystonia, akathisia, and oculogyric crisis. Stopping the droperidol (Inapsine) and administration of intravenous diphenhydramine hydrochloride (Benadryl) rapidly reverses the extrapyramidal symptoms and must be followed by oral doses for 24 to 48 hours. Diphenidol (Vontrol) is an oral preparation that appears to exert a specific antivertigo effect on the vestibular nuclei. It is also a potent antiemetic. Due to the 0.5% incidence of visual and auditory hallucinations, it is recommended that therapy be initiated in the hospital and monitored for 3 to 4 days before discharge. If hallucinations occur they usually resolve within 3 days after stopping the medication. Once an effective dosage is achieved, and no hallucinations are encountered, routine follow-up should include periodic complete blood count to check for blood dyscrasia.

In addition to pharmacologic therapies, many patients with Meniere's disease require psychological support to help cope with the frustrations and changes brought about by their medical condition. This can be accomplished with individual counselors, extra time spent during office visits, or often most successfully with support groups composed of patients who share the same condition. One such group is a national program called The Meniere's Network (c/o The EAR Foundation, 2000 Church St., Nashville, TN 37236). This network offers a quarterly publication that provides information on Meniere's disease and updates on available treatments, as well as regional support groups and information sources. Providing patients access to this type of resource can have a positive impact on their sense of control over their disease and their compliance with prescribed therapy.

The vertigo suffered by the majority of Meniere's patients can usually be controlled using dietary sodium restriction and diuretics in combination with vestibular suppressants when indicated. Those patients in whom the vertigo becomes disabling by virtue of increased severity or frequency of attacks, in spite of maximal medical therapy, would then be considered candidates for surgical intervention in an attempt to control vertigo. The available surgical options are covered in a subsequent section of this chapter.

A separate group of Meniere's disease patients warrants discussion at this point: patients with Meniere's disease affecting both ears. The same measures used to control unilateral disease are also effective, but when symptoms become disabling it is difficult to positively identify the offending ear. This inability to identify the troublesome ear eliminates many surgical options in treating disabling vertigo. In this situation, bilateral vestibular ablation can be considered as a treatment alternative. Parenteral (usually intramuscular) administration of streptomycin is undertaken in the hospital, closely monitoring the patient's hearing and vestibular function. When symptoms of ataxia develop during treatment, daily caloric examinations are done until nystagmus is no longer produced with stimulation by ice water. In addition to monitoring caloric response, screening audiometry is done to minimize risk of hearing loss during the ablation. Once ablation has been completed, patients are usually freed of the severe vertigo attacks but are left with some chronic unsteadiness. The most common manifestation of bilateral vestibular ablation is the symptom of oscillopsia. Interestingly, the vestibule exhibits some capability of recuperating from this type of metabolic assault, and patients who have received streptomycin ablation may require repeat administration for recurrent symptoms (often accompanied by a return of response on ice water caloric testing).

Labyrinthitis

The treatment of viral labyrinthitis centers around controlling vertigo. This is accomplished with the use of the vestibular suppressants discussed in the section on medical management of Meniere's disease. In addition, bed rest is very helpful early on in the course of the disease. Attention must be paid to the patient's overall fluid status since fluid loss from prolonged vomiting may necessitate intravenous replacement and electrolyte management. Usually the first 24 to 72 hours are the most symptomatic for the patient. After the most severe vertigo has passed, then ambulation may resume with assistance; independent ambulation may be achieved over the next few days. Once at this level, patients should be encouraged to diminish their use of vestibular suppressants to accelerate the process of central compensation. To further speed up the process of recuperation, vestibular conditioning exercises (i.e., Cawthorne exercises) challenge the compensatory mechanisms of the central nervous system, stimulating adaptation. The symptomatology is usually self-limited to a course of approximately 6 weeks.

Vestibular Neuronitis

The vertigo of vestibular neuronitis is controlled in much the same manner as in labyrinthitis, with vestibular suppressants. The tendency for recurrent vertigo to occur may result in the need to treat periodically for relapses. There is some theoretic support for the use of a tapering burst dose of corticosteroids, but their efficacy has not been conclusively demonstrated. It is often difficult to diagnose which ear is diseased, but when it can be identified, surgery may be an option if symptoms become debilitating.

Benign Paroxysmal Positional Vertigo

This usually self-limited disorder is best treated with vestibular conditioning exercises. The patient is instructed to assume repeatedly the positions that bring on the symptoms in an effort to fatigue the response and stimulate more rapid central compensation. The use of vestibular suppressants may actually slow down the process of central compensation and are usually not necessary. The period of recovery from this condition is usually 6 weeks to 6 months. However, in some patients, usually the more elderly, the symptoms persist in spite of compliance with vestibular conditioning exercises. In these patients, vestibular suppressants may be useful. Recent experiences with astemizole (Hismanal) shows promise for reliable symptom control in patients with BPPV. For more severe symptoms unresponsive to exercises and medical treatment, surgical options are available for relief.

Autoimmune Vestibulopathy

Since autoimmune vestibulopathy usually affects both ears, therapy is almost exclusively medical. Vestibular suppressants are most useful in controlling the more severe exacerbations of vertigo. The main thrust of therapy would be directed at the underlying autoimmune condition. The use of corticosteroids and some cytotoxic agents (cytoxan, methotrexate) has been shown to provide relief in some patients. There is some newer evidence to suggest that serum plasmapheresis may play a more prominent role in controlling this disease in the future. The natural history of the disease leads to eventual bilateral vestibular ablation, caused by the disease process. This end result is almost inevitable unless the underlying process can be arrested with treatment or arrests spontaneously.

Vascular Vertigo

Since the symptoms of vertigo attributable to vascular etiologies stem, for the most part, from compromised circulation to the central nervous system, the basic goal of treatment is to improve blood supply. In vaso–occlusive disease, medications with antiplatelet activity are the first line of treatment. Aspirin taken in low doses inhibits platelet aggregation and diminishes the likelihood of an infarction. By this action it may improve circulation in low flow areas. Vasodilators such as dipyridamole (Persantine) may be useful in improving circulation. Rarely are symptoms so severe that the use of anticoagulants such as heparin or warfarin (Coumadin) is indicated.

In those patients with posterior circulation migraine, therapy should be directed at preventing or aborting attacks. This is accomplished in the same manner as with classic migraine. Prevention may be accomplished by the use of beta-blockers such as propranolol (Inderal), or by employing methysergide (Sansert). There is a great risk of serious side effects, such as pleuropulmonary and retroperitoneal fibrosis, with methysergide, and it should be reserved for those patients with frequent and severe vascular headaches/vertigo that have been uncontrollable on other medications. Ergotamine tartrate, usually in combination with caffeine (Cafergot), is highly useful in aborting attacks early in their evolution. These preparations come in both oral and suppository preparations. Patients with migraine equivalents should be referred to a neurologist for management, unless the clinician is familiar with the management of vascular headaches.

SURGICAL MANAGEMENT OF VERTIGO

Meniere's Disease

Considerable controversy still exists regarding the proper surgical management of those Meniere's patients who have failed medical therapy. This segment discusses the currently accepted procedures and some of their merits and reviews published success rates. The first group of procedures includes those designed to control vertigo and preserve hearing.

Endolymphatic sac surgery was first proposed in 1926 by Portmann when he described endolymphatic sac decompression. After falling out of favor for some time, endolymphatic sac surgery was revived by William House in the early 1960s with the addition of endolymph shunting. A variety of procedures designed to drain the sac evolved. Some sought to shunt the endolymphatic fluid into the subarachnoid space, while others shunted it into the mastoid. Simple silastic sheating, tubing, and complex unidirectional valved shunts have all been used in recent years. Reported success rates for controlling vertigo with endolymphatic shunt surgery range from 60% to 80%. Silverstein recently suggested that there is little difference between these reported successes and the natural history of symptom resolution in medically treated patients. A controversial study in 1981 by Thomsen, et al. compared simple mastoidectomy to endolymphatic sac decompression and drainage. They found little difference between these two groups and ascribed much of the perceived postoperative improvement in symptoms to the placebo effect. Hence the efficacy of this technique has come under some question.

Sacculotomy, in one form or another, has been proposed by a variety of authors as a method of relieving the pressure build-up in the endolymphatic chamber. In the mid 1960s Fick described sacculotomy for relief of vertigo attributable to Meniere's disease. Cody then reported his Tack operation in 1967, which effected an automatic sacculotomy when the saccule became dilated. These procedures faded from popularity as a high percentage of patients suffered severe sensorineural hearing loss as a result of surgery. It was not until 1982 that Schuknecht revived interest in saccular decompression with his report of the cochleosacculotomy. The long-term success rates for this procedure are not yet available, and there have been reported occurrences of dead ears as a result of the surgery. Silverstein in 1984 reported significant hearing loss in 50% in patients undergoing cochleosacculotomy. He did, however, point out its advantages: ease of performance, utility in elderly patients as a first procedure under local anesthesia, and little risk other than hearing loss.

The current treatment most successful in controlling medically recalcitrant vertigo is the vestibular nerve section. This procedure is indicated in individuals with serviceable hearing in whom maximal medical therapy has been unsuccessful in controlling vertigo. Serviceable hearing is considered to be hearing loss that could be successfully rehabilitated with a hearing aid. Some patients may not yet have a significant hearing loss in spite of severe vertigo symptoms. Success rates in the range of 90% to 95% have been reported by numerous authors. There are a variety of routes available to the surgeon undertaking a vestibular nerve section.

Dandy, in 1928, described the suboccipital (also known as retrosigmoid) approach for sectioning the eighth cranial nerve as a method of controlling vertigo in Meniere's patients. This procedure was not a hearing preservation operation in his original description. However, with modern refinements this approach, with the selective sectioning of the vestibular branch of the eighth cranial nerve, provides reliable control of vertigo with little operative risk to hearing. The retrolabyrinthine and middle fossa approaches popularized by House, Fisch, and Glasscock in the 1970s and early 1980s also provide reliable results but are technically more difficult, and do not provide as generous exposure to the cerebellopontine angle as the suboccipital approach in the event of accidental vascular injury. For the latter reasons, the suboccipital or retrosigmoid approach is most commonly used for selective vestibular nerve section.

An important improvement in the safety of vestibular nerve section relating to the preservation of hearing and facial nerve function is the availability of intraoperative monitoring of these nerves. Electromyographic monitoring of facial nerve activity provides the surgeon with a highly sensitive means of monitoring undue facial nerve irritation. This irritation may be mechanical, thermodynamic, or electrical. Due to the extreme sensitivity of this monitoring technique, the surgeon is often alerted before any permanent damage is sustained by the nerve. With regard to monitoring hearing function, intraoperative use of brainstem-evoked response audiometry helps the surgeon ensure an adequate vestibular nerve section while at the same time indicating any undesired cochlear nerve impingement. As a further extension of this monitoring technique, monitoring electrodes are available that can be placed directly on the cochlear branch of the eighth nerve during the procedure to warn of injury. These advances have reduced the morbidity associated with this surgery.

The next group of procedures are considered "destructive," since hearing is sacrificed in the effort to control vertigo. These procedures are recommended in those individuals with nonserviceable hearing. The hearing loss in these patients is so severe that they could not fruitfully wear a hearing aid in the involved ear. The least invasive of these is the transmeatal labyrinthectomy as described by Schuknecht in 1956 and Cawthorne in 1957. This procedure allows removal of all the important neuroepithelial structures of the membranous labyrinth via an enlargement of the oval window. The transmeatal route eliminates the need for mastoidectomy and reduces operative time. Its disadvantages are the limited exposure and the possibility of incomplete removal of the neuroepithelial elements and return of vertigo.

Transmastoid or translabyrinthine labyrinthectomy provides a total removal of the vestibular neuroepithelial elements and has a demonstrated success rate of 95% for elimination of vertigo. Like transmeatal labyrinthectomy it requires general anesthetic, primarily to avoid patient movement during the acute destruction of the labyrinth. The semicircular canals are removed along with their ampullae, allowing extraction of the cristae. The main chamber of the vestibule is opened and the saccule and utricle avulsed with their maculae. An extension of this surgery is the translabyrinthine vestibular nerve section, shown to eliminate vertigo in 98% of cases. After the vestibule is opened, the internal auditory canal is partially skeletonized, allowing the exposure of the eighth cranial nerve in the canal. The nerve is then partially resected along with Scarpa's ganglion. This procedure is more risky, since the facial nerve is at greater risk and CSF leak may occur as the dura of the internal auditory canal must be opened to perform the surgery. This increased risk does not seem warranted for so slight an increase (3%) in the success rate.

Benign Paroxysmal Positional Vertigo

When vestibular conditioning exercises fail to control the symptoms of BPPV, there are two surgical options. The first is transmeatal posterior ampullary nerve section (also known as singular neurectomy). In this procedure the posterior ampullary nerve is identified in the singular canal inferior and posterior to the round window via the transmeatal approach. Once identified, it is sectioned and the singular canal obliterated with bone wax. This technique is challenging and has the associated risk of cochlear injury during the exposure of the singular canal. Vestibular nerve section is the other available option and has been discussed earlier. Its disadvantages are that it requires a craniectomy and has potential CNS complications.

Perilymph Fistula

Considerable controversy persists surrounding the frequency with which perilymph fistulas are found at surgery. Clearly, however, there are those patients in whom the history, symptomatology, and diagnostic evaluation strongly suggest the possibility of perilymphatic fistula. In these patients, surgical management consists of middle ear exploration and packing of the oval and round window areas. The materials chosen to pack these areas include fat, Gelfoam, and areolar and/or fibrous tissue. These areas are packed whether or not a clear-cut fistula is demonstrated. Reported success rates for this treatment vary and likely reflect some element of variable patient selection.

Vascular Loop Syndrome

As Janetta popularized vascular decompression of the trigeminal nerve via the suboccipital approach for control of trigeminal neuralgia, there is growing momentum for vascular decompression of the eighth cranial nerve as a method of controlling vertigo in patients with vascular loop syndrome. Vestibular nerve section has been demonstrated as an effective means of relieving vertigo in patients with documented vascular loops. Further characterization of this syndrome needs to take place, and a clear-cut relationship between the presence of vascular loops and the symptom of vertigo, with or without hearing loss, has to be established. The retrolabyrinthine and suboccipital approaches are the same as those used to perform vestibular nerve section and have the same attendant risks. The efficacy of neurovascular decompression alone has yet to be conclusively demonstrated and is still an area requiring further study.

SUMMARY

This chapter covered a wide range of medical and surgical treatment of both peripheral and central causes of vertigo. The majority of these treatments can effectively be provided by the otolaryngologist. More advanced forms of surgical and even medical therapy warrant the involvement of a neurotologist, and occasionally a neurosurgeon or neurologist. It is hoped that an improved understanding of the disease process and its treatment will allow the clinican to provide the best level of care possible for his/her patients.

SUGGESTED READING

1. Jackson CG, Glasscock ME, Davis WE, Hughes GB, Sismanis A. Medical management of Meniere's disease. *Ann Otol Rhinol Laryngol,* 1981;90:142.
2. Wilson WR, Schuknecht HS. Update on the use of streptomycin therapy for Meniere's disease. *Am J Otol* 1980;2:108.
3. Brandt T, Daroff RB. Physical therapy for benign paroxysmal positional vertigo. *Arch Otolaryngol* 1980;106:484.
4. Luetje CM. Theoretical and practical implications for plasmapheresis in autoimmune inner ear disease. *Laryngoscope* 1989;99:1137.
5. Portmann G. The saccus endolymphaticus and an operation for draining the same for relief of vertigo. *J Laryngol Otol* 1927;42:809.
6. House WF. Subarachnoid shunt for drainage of endolymphatic hydrops. *Laryngoscope* 1962;72:713.
7. Silverstein H, Smouha E, Jones R. Natural history versus surgery for Meniere's disease. *Otolaryngol Head Neck Surg* 1989;100:6.
8. Thomsen J, et al. Placebo effect in surgery for Meniere's disease: a double-

blind, placebo-controlled study on endolymphatic sac shunt surgery. *Arch Otolaryngol* 1981;107:271.

9. Fick IA, Decompression of the labyrinth. *Arch Otolaryngol* 1964;79:447.
10. Cody DT. The tack operation for endolymphatic hydrops. *Laryngoscope* 1969;79:1737.
11. Schuknecht HF. Cochleosacculotomy for Meniere's disease: theory, technique, and results. *Laryngoscope* 1982;92:853.
12. Silverstein H. Hyman S, Silverstein D. Cochleosacculotomy. *Otolaryngol Head and Neck Surg* 1984;92:63.
13. Dandy WE. Meniere's disease: its diagnosis and a method of treatment. *Arch Surg* 1928;16:1127.
14. House WF. Surgical exposure of the internal auditory canal and its contents through the middle cranial fossa. *Laryngoscope* 1961;71:1363.
15. Fisch U. Vestibular and cochlear neurectomy. *Trans Am Acad Ophthalmol Otolaryngol* 1977;78:252.
16. Glasscock ME. Middle fossa approach to the temporal bone. *Arch Otolaryngol,* 1969;90:41.
17. Schuknecht HF. Ablation therapy for the relief of Meniere's disease. *Laryngoscope* 1956;66:859.
18. Cawthorne T. Membranous labyrinthectomy via the oval window for Meniere's disease. *J Laryngol Otol* 1957;71:524.
19. Glasscock ME, Hughes GB, Davis WE, Jackson CG. Labyrinthectomy versus middle fossa vestibular nerve section in Meniere's disease. *Ann Otol Rhinol Laryngol* 1980;89:318.
20. Gacek RR. Transection of the posterior ampullary nerve for the relief of benign paroxysmal positional vertigo. *Ann Otol* 1974;83:596.
21. Wiet RJ, Schramm DR, Kazan RP. Retrolabyrinthine approach and vascular loop. *Laryngoscope* 1989;99:1035.
22. Kraus B. *Complete guide to sodium.* New York: Signet Book, NAL Penguin, Inc., 1987.
23. Kraus B. *Sodium guide to brand name and basic foods.* New York: Signet Book, NAL Penguin, Inc., 1985.

6

Case Studies

Chapter 6 reviews a series of case histories designed to illustrate some of the more common causes of vertigo. While comprehensive, it is not meant to list or set forth an example of every possible etiology known to produce the symptom of vertigo. An attempt has been made to document actual case histories from the files of The Otology Group. Some of these patients were seen before the advent of computerized axial tomography (CT) or magnetic resonance imaging (MRI) scanners and they are of particular interest from an historical viewpoint.

Representative audiograms, auditory brainstem response (ABR), and electronystagmography (ENG), as well as CT and MRI images are included with most case histories.

CASE 1.   MENIERE'S DISEASE

J.B., a 48-year-old woman, presented in April of 1989 with 5-year history of monthly vertiginous episodes lasting approximately 2 days with associated fluctuation in hearing on the left. The episodes were exacerbated by increased salt intake and had become nearly continuous during the preceding 5 weeks. Her past surgical history was significant for removal of a middle ear adenoma 10 years before with ossicular reconstruction.

The physical examination was within normal limits except for left mild posterior tympanic membrane retraction.

An audiogram (Fig. 1) showed normal hearing on the right with an air conduction average of 0 dB and 100% speech discrimination. The speech reception threshold (SRT) on the right was 25 dB with a

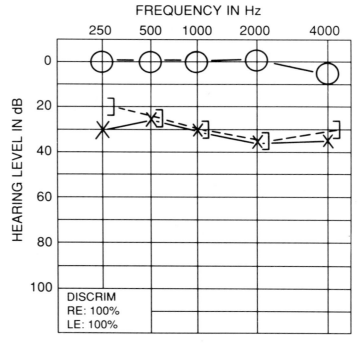

FIG. 1. Audiogram, case 1, J. B. (Meniere's disease).

100% discrimination score and an air bone gap of 20 dB in all frequencies tested.

An ENG was grossly normal and the ABR showed normal wave progression bilaterally.

CT and MRI scans were normal. She underwent a left retrosigmoid vestibular nerve section on May 10, 1989. A good cleavage plane was seen between the vestibular and cochlear portions of the nerve. Her hospital stay was uneventful, and on her 1 month follow-up visit she complained of only mild unsteadiness. Her hearing was maintained at her preoperative level. She has had no further vertigo, and her hearing has remained stable.

Comment: This rather typical case of Meniere's disease did not respond to medical management. The retrosigmoid vestibular nerve section is a reliable surgical procedure for dealing with medical failure.

CASE 2.   MENIERE'S DISEASE

R.H., a 50-year-old man, presented in April 1989 with complaints of dizziness and fluctuating left hearing loss and tinnitus. The vertiginous episodes were exacerbated by lying down and lasted approximately 1 hour. He complained of constant unsteadiness and veered to the left when walking. The patient had been diagnosed 10 years previously as having Meniere's disease. He had undergone a right endolymphatic sac decompression 8 years previously, followed by a total right labyrinthectomy the following year for persistent symptoms. A CT scan of the head had been normal at the time of surgery.

On physical examination the standing Romberg was within normal limits, although he had an unsteady gait. The remainder of the physical examination was normal.

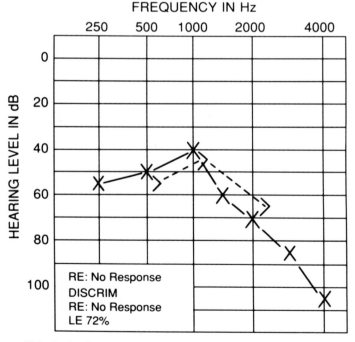

FIG. 2. Audiogram, case 2, R. H. (Meniere's disease).

The audiogram showed no hearing in the right ear. There was a left high-frequency sensorineural hearing loss with a speech reception threshold (SRT) of 50 dB and a discrimination score of 72% (Fig. 2).

An electronystagmogram (ENG) indicated a left reduced vestibular response (report, Fig. 3). The ABR was within normal limits on the left with no response on the right secondary to the profound loss (Fig. 4). An MRI scan was normal.

The patient was treated with Dyazide (hydrochlorothiazide–triameterene) and a low salt diet for Meniere's disease in his only hearing ear. Streptomycin therapy was recommended by the referring physician, to which the patient has responded well.

Comment: Streptomycin injection following the Schuknecht protocol is an effective way to treat Meniere's disease in an only hearing ear.

ELECTRONYSTAGMOGRAPHY REPORT

Case 2: RH

1.	**Spont. Nystagmus**	-- _X_ NEG ___ RB ___LB
2.	**Gaze Nystagmus**	-- _X_ NEG ___ RB ___LB
3.	**Optokinetic**	-- _X_ SYM ___ ASYM
4.	**Eye Tracking**	-- _X_ I ___ II ___ III ___ IV
5.	**Positionals'**	-- _X_ NEG ___ RB ___ LB ___ DIR CHG _____

BITHERMAL CALORIC STIMULATION

$R-44^0$	___ WNL	___ Slightly Reduced	_X_ No Response
$L-44^0$	___ WNL	_X_ Slightly Reduced	___ No Response
$R-30^0$	___ WNL	___ Slightly Reduced	_X_ No Response
$L-30^0$	___ WNL	___ Slightly Reduced	_X_ No Response
	_____ %	_____ Unilateral Weakness	
	_____ %	_____ Directional Preponderance	

COMMENT: No response right consistent with past history of labyrinthectomy. Reduced response on the left compared to normal.

CLINICAL IMPRESSION: Reduced vestibular response, left. No response, right.

FIG. 3. Electronystagmography (ENG), case 2. R. H. (Meniere's disease).

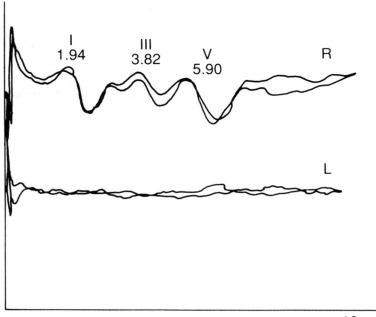

FIG. 4. Auditory brainstem response (ABR), case 2, R. H. (Meniere's disease).

CASE 3. VESTIBULAR NEURONITIS

K.O., a 67-year-old woman, was seen in April of 1989 complaining of acute vertigo following an episode of influenza in February of 1989. The initial attack was very severe, lasting 4 to 5 days, and was associated with nausea and vomiting. In the ensuing 2 months she experienced vertigo with position change.

Physical examination was normal. She had a long-standing bilateral sensorineural hearing loss (Fig. 5).

ENG (Fig. 6) was non-localizing and her ABR and MRI scan were normal (Figs. 7, 8).

She was started on Valium (diazepam) 5 mg and Robinul (glycopyrrolate) 2 mg to be taken when she experienced vertigo. Her symptoms gradually subsided and she no longer requires labyrinthine sedatives.

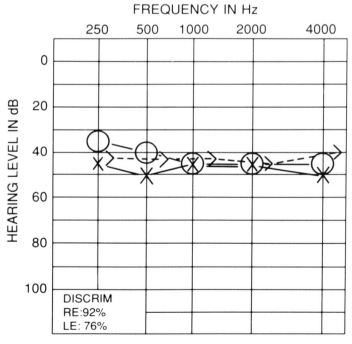

FIG. 5. Audiogram, case 3. K. O. (vestibular neuronitis).

Comment: This patient experienced a typical vestibular neuronitis or viral labyrinthitis following an episode of influenza. These are self-limiting vestibular dysfunctions in which there is usually a reduction of function in one labyrinth on ENG. After the initial episode, the patient is left with positional vertigo that generally responds to labyrinthine sedatives such as Valium.

ELECTRONYSTAGMOGRAPHY REPORT

Case 3: KO

1. **Spont. Nystagmus** -- ___ NEG _X_ RB ___LB

2. **Gaze Nystagmus** -- _X_ NEG ___ RB ___LB

3. **Optokinetic** -- ___ SYM _X_ ASYM

4. **Eye Tracking** -- _X_ I ___ II ___ III ___ IV

5. **Positionals** -- ___ NEG _X_ RB ___ LB ___ DIR CHG _____

BITHERMAL CALORIC STIMULATION

R-44^0	_X_ WNL	___ Slightly Reduced	___ No Response
L-44^0	_X_ WNL	___ Slightly Reduced	___ No Response
R-30^0	_X_ WNL	___ Slightly Reduced	___ No Response
L-30^0	_X_ WNL	___ Slightly Reduced	___ No Response
	_1_ %	_RT_ Unilateral Weakness	
	_11_ %	_RT_ Directional Preponderance	

COMMENT: Caloric responses are within normal limits, but there is evidence of spontaneous and positional nystagmus.

CLINICAL IMPRESSION: Abnormal recording, nonlocalizing.

FIG. 6. Electronystagmography (ENG), case 3, K. O. (vestibular neuronitis).

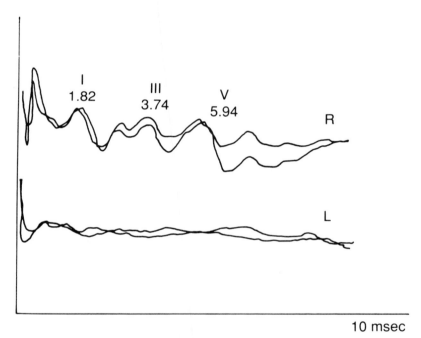

FIG. 7. Auditory brainstem response (ABR), case 3, K. O. (vestibular neu-ronitis).

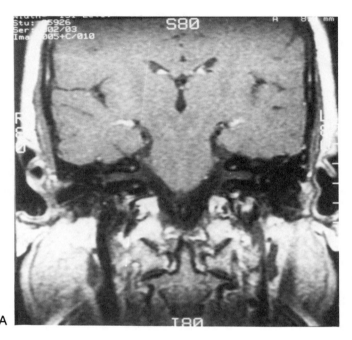

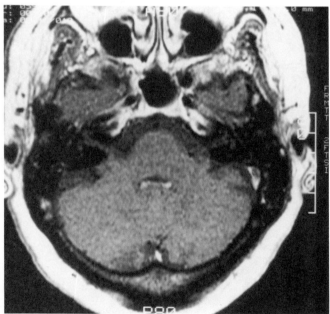

FIG. 8. A: MRI, normal coronal view of internal auditory canals, case 3, K. O. **B:** MRI, normal axial view of internal auditory canals, case 3, K. O.

CASE 4. ACOUSTIC NEUROMA

L.C. is a 40-year-old man who presented with the chief complaint of hearing loss in the left ear and vertigo over a 6-month period. More recently, he had noticed tinnitus in the left ear.

His otologic examination was normal except for the left-sided hearing loss. The audiogram revealed normal hearing in the right ear and a mild sensorineural loss in the left ear. Speech discrimination scores were excellent bilaterally (Fig. 9).

ENG revealed essentially equal caloric responses. ABR, however, was notable in that no response could be observed on stimulation of the left ear (Fig. 10).

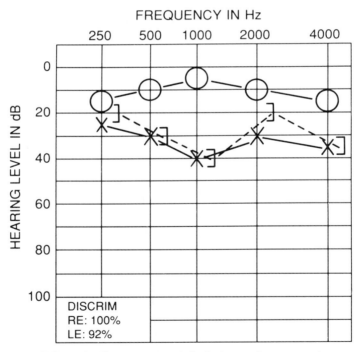

FIG. 9. Audiogram, case 4, L. C. (acoustic neuroma).

A gadolinium-enhanced MRI was obtained and demonstrated a 1.7-cm mass in the cerebellopontine angle extending into the internal auditory canal (Fig. 11).

The patient underwent a translabyrinthine resection of this mass, which proved to be an acoustic neuroma. The facial nerve was preserved, and facial nerve function appeared excellent at the time of discharge from the hospital.

Comment.   While some patients with acoustic nerve tumors do not complain of vertigo because of the slow growth rate and the process of vestibular accommodation, this complaint does not rule out a tumor. Anyone with a unilateral sensorineural hearing loss and vertigo should have an MRI with gadolinium.

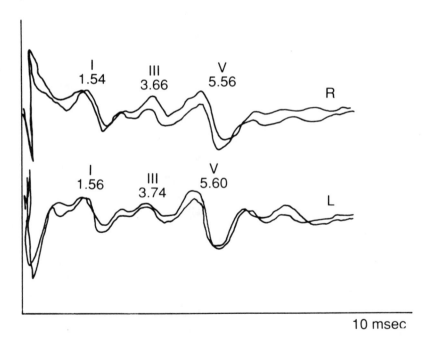

FIG. 10. Auditory brainstem response (ABR), case 4. L. C. (acoustic neuroma).

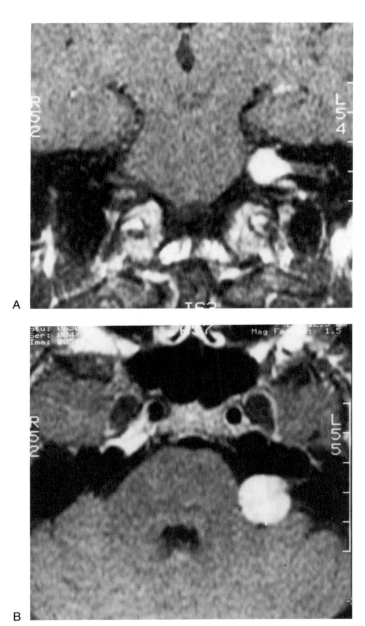

FIG. 11. A: MRI, Coronal view, left. Acoustic neuroma in internal auditory canals and CPA, case 4. L. C. **B:** MRI, Axial view left. Acoustic neuroma, case 4. L. C.

CASE 5.   CENTRAL NERVOUS SYSTEM TUMOR

R.N., a 27-year-old man, presented in October 1988 with complaints of two episodes of dizziness lasting several minutes during
the preceding 3 months. He had occasional right-sided tinnitus, but
no hearing loss or aural fullness. The patient did have occasional
mild numbness of the right arm and leg lasting a few minutes.

The physical examination was within normal limits.

An audiogram (Fig. 12) was normal, with an SRT of 0 dB and
100% discrimination on the right and a 5 dB SRT with 100% discrimination on the left.

The ABR was within normal limits on the left (Fig. 13), but there
were morphologic abnormalities on the right, with a marked II–III
delay consistent with retrocochlear pathology.

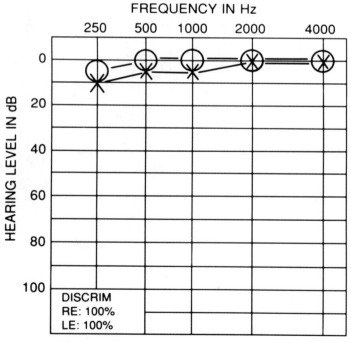

FIG. 12. Audiogram, case 5. R. N. (CNS tumor).

MRI axial and coronal T_1-weighted (Figs. 14 and 15) showed a nonenhancing 1.2×3.2-cm mixed density mass in the right cerebellopontine angle.

The patient underwent a right suboccipital excision of the mass. The tumor was macerated and cystic in nature, invading the pons. A frozen section was consistent with an astrocytoma. Each cyst was widely fenestrated, decompressing the cerebellopontine angle. Due to obvious invasion into the substance of the pons the tumor was not completely resected, and all cranial nerves were spared.

Comment: ABR is valuable as a method of screening patients for central nervous system disease. Abnormal ABR findings should be followed by an MRI with gadolinium.

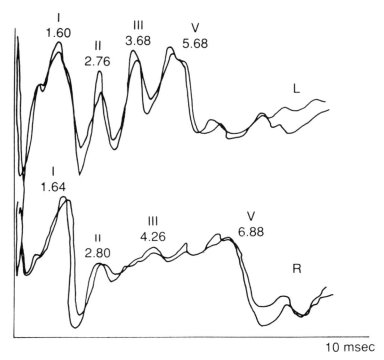

10 msec

FIG. 13. Auditory brainstem response (ABR), case 5. R. N. (CNS tumor).

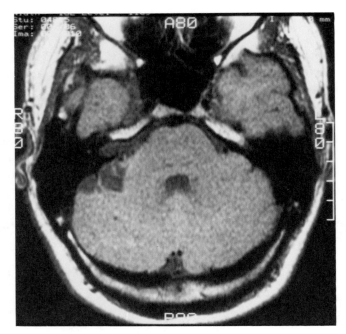

FIG. 14. MRI, axial view right. Cerebellar astrocytoma, case 5.

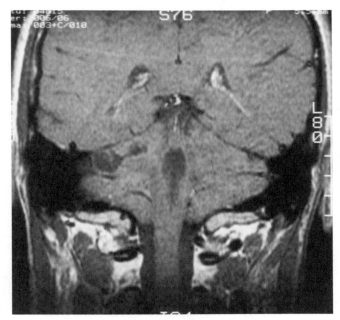

FIG. 15. MRI, coronal view right. Cerebellar astrocytoma, case 5.

CASE 6.   CENTRAL NERVOUS SYSTEM TUMOR

W.W., a 42-year-old woman, presented in May of 1977 with a 2 to 3 year history of episodic vertigo and nausea. She had noticed fluctuation of her left hearing with aural fullness and left-sided tinnitus. She had experienced intermittent occipital headaches during the same period.

The physical examination was within normal limits except for a positive Romberg test with mild gait ataxia.

An audiogram was normal (Fig. 16), and an ENG elicited an extremely strong gaze nystagmus. For this reason calorics were not performed. Petrous pyramid X-ray views were normal.

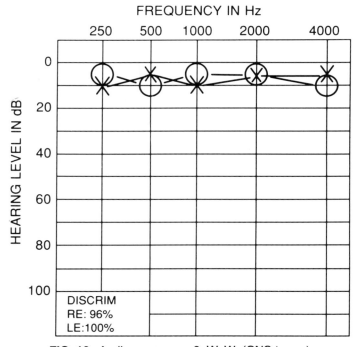

FIG. 16. Audiogram, case 6, W. W. (CNS tumor).

An ABR was normal on the left, but there was no response on the right (Fig. 17). Because of the abnormal ABR and the patient's ataxia a CT scan was ordered. This study revealed a 3-cm cerebello-pontine angle mass on the right side. There was some question whether this was an acoustic tumor or some unusual lesion of the angle.

Because of the presenting symptoms, a diagnosis of left-sided Meniere's disease was entertained, and the patient was started on a low salt diet and Dyazide. Valium and Robinul were to be used with attacks of vertigo.

On August 17, 1977 a combined translabyrinthine–suboccipital approach to the right cerebellopontine angle was performed. The tumor was continuous with the fourth ventricle, and pathologic evaluation revealed it to be a papilloma of the choroid plexus arising from the ventricle. A small piece of tumor was left in the ventricle be-

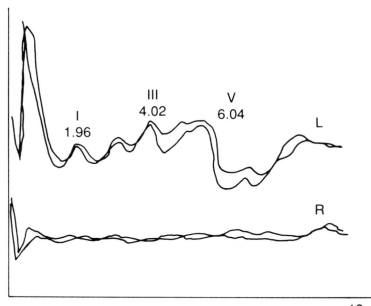

10 msec

FIG. 17. ABR, case 6, W. W. (CNS tumor).

cause the neurosurgeon did not feel comfortable in removing it through the combined approach.

Later, in October of 1977, the neurosurgeon went back through a midline approach and removed the small amount of residual tumor from the fourth ventricle.

The patient later developed a cerebrospinal fluid (CSF) leak that required surgical closure. Two months later she came into the hospital with acute hydrocephalus that required a ventriculo–peritoneal shunt.

She subsequently did well and required no further treatment.

Comment: The authors have no good explanation for her left-sided symptoms of fluctuating hearing loss, fullness, and tinnitus. The symptoms cleared after her tumor removal.

This case was one of the first in the authors' practice in which the CT scanner was used to establish the correct diagnosis. The ABR played a vital role because the abnormal tracing prompted the CT scan.

CASE 7.   MULTIPLE SCLEROSIS

J.S., a 47-year-old woman with a 2-year history of disequilibrium and falling to the left, presented in December, 1973 with a recently diagnosed left-sided hearing loss on routine physical exam. Past medical history was significant for retrobulbar neuronitis of the left eye 17 years before evaluation that had been treated with steroids and that resolved with resultant blurring of central left vision.

The physical examination was normal except for falling to the left on Romberg evaluation.

An audiogram (Fig. 18) was performed, which showed an SRT of 0 dB with 100% discrimination on the right. There was a high-frequency sensorineural hearing loss on the left, with an SRT of 4 dB and speech discrimination of 88%.

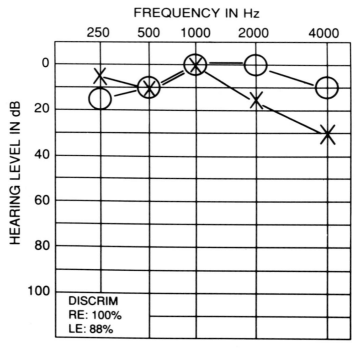

FIG. 18. Audiogram, case 7. J. S. (multiple sclerosis).

The ABR showed abnormal brainstem transmission bilaterally (Fig. 19). The waveforms were delayed, and there were morphologic abnormalities. X-ray films of the petrous pyramid were within normal limits. With these findings the patient was referred for a neurologic evaluation with a strong suspicion of multiple sclerosis. She subsequently died from this disease 10 years later.

Comment: Her presenting symptoms were difficult to explain on the basis of an inner problem. The first tip-off that she might have MS was the abnormal ABR. This patient was seen long before MRI was available. Currently the MRI is extremely helpful in confirming the diagnosis of MS.

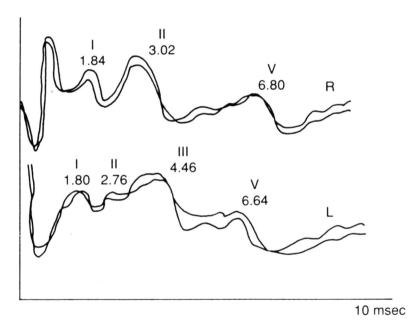

10 msec

FIG. 19. Auditory brainstem response (ABR), case 7, J. S. (multiple sclerosis).

CASE 8. NEUROSYPHILIS

A.P., a 19-year-old man was referred in November 1977 for a second opinion. Two months prior to evaluation the patient had awakened acutely vertiginous with a left-sided hearing loss. The vertiginous symptoms resolved, with the patient remaining unsteady, and he began to notice increasing left-sided tinnitus. The hearing had subjectively fluctuated, and a previous audiogram showed a moderately severe sensorineural hearing loss in both high and low frequencies, with speech discrimination of 32% on the left. The past history was significant for a 5-year history of slowly progressive high-frequency loss on the right. A fluorescent treponemal antibody-absorption test (FTA-ABS) had been reactive, and the patient had been treated with appropriate therapy consisting of Bicillin (penicillin G benzathine) injections and prednisone.

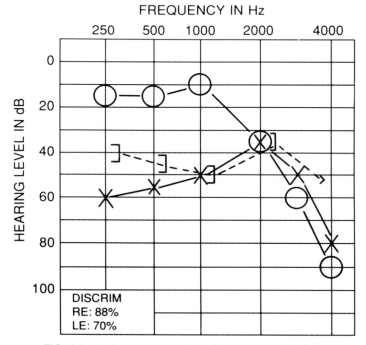

FIG. 20. Audiogram, case 8, A. P. (neurosyphilis).

At this visit, the physical examination was within normal limits.

An audiogram showed bilateral sensorineural hearing with an SRT of 20 dB and speech discrimination of 88% on the right. The left SRT was 47 dB, and discrimination had improved to 70% (Fig. 20). CT scan and posterior fossa myelogram was ordered to rule out a possible acoustic neuroma, but they were within normal limits.

Repeat serologic tests for syphilis were reactive.

The patient had been adequately treated for neurosyphilis with antibiotics and steroids; therefore no further therapy was considered. The symptom of unsteadiness was improved with diazepam as needed. The patient was told that he might require steroids from time to time in the future.

Comment: Neurosyphilis is not a common problem today, but it still occurs. With bilateral, fluctuating hearing loss and vertigo, an FTA-ABS should be an integral part of the evaluation.

CASE 9.   VASCULAR INSUFFICIENCY—
CAROTID OCCLUSION

C.P., a 60-year-old woman, presented in January, 1989 with an 8-day history of constant unsteadiness, vertigo, and acute, severe, left-sided hearing loss. There was fullness in the left ear and transient pulsatile tinnitus. The patient also experienced mild left-sided numbness at the onset of symptoms that resolved after 2 hours. Her past medical history was significant for a transient ischemic attack (TIA) involving the left hemisphere and two previous myocardial infarctions (MI).

The physical examination was significant for positive Romberg test to the left and left-sided past pointing. There was also diminished carotid pulsation on the right.

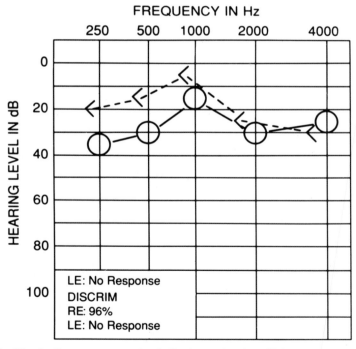

FIG. 21. Audiogram, case 9. C. P. (vascular insufficiency—carotid occlusion).

An audiogram showed an SRT of 30 dB on the right with 96% discrimination. The left ear was essentially anacousic (Fig. 21).

A four-vessel arteriogram was obtained that showed 95% stenosis of the right internal carotid artery at the level of the bifurcation (Fig. 22) and complete obstruction of the left internal carotid artery.

The patient subsequently underwent a right carotid endarterectomy performed by the neurosurgical service without complications.

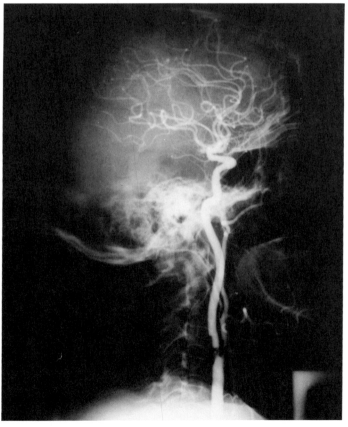

A

FIG. 22. A: Arteriogram, lateral view right. Internal and external carotid stenosis, case 9. C. P.

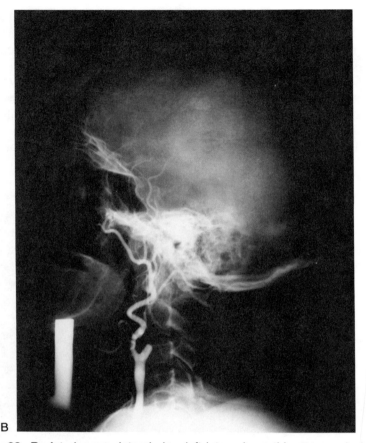

B

FIG. 22. B: Arteriogram, lateral view left internal carotid artery occlusion, case 9. C. P.

The vertiginous symptoms subsided postoperatively. Prior to discharge, an MRI scan with gadolinium was obtained to rule out a concurrent cerebellopontine angle tumor. This was negative.

The patient was doing well at 6-month follow-up, with strong temporal pulses bilaterally. There were no further episodes of vertigo and only minimal unsteadiness. She also had noted a subjective improvement of hearing on the left, which has not yet been confirmed by audiogram.

Comment: Patients with a history of coronary disease and episodes of TIA who experience vertigo should have at least a Doppler of the carotids, and if that is abnormal an arteriogram is in order.

CASE 10. VASCULAR INSUFFIENCY — SMALL VESSEL DISEASE

M.M., a 81-year-old woman, presented in May of 1989 with a 2-year history of constant unsteadiness. During the preceding 3 months she had experienced true vertiginous episodes lasting 4 to 5 seconds that were initiated by head rotation and lying down. She denied change in hearing or tinnitus, and had been previously placed on Persantine (dipyridamole), Pavabid (papaverine hydrochloride), and Meclizine (HCL) without resolution of her symptoms. A recent MRI scan and carotid doppler studies were within normal limits.

Physical exam was normal except for a mildly positive Romberg with a drift to the right.

An audiogram (Fig. 23) showed bilateral sensorineural hearing loss predominantly in the high frequencies. SRTs were 30 dB on the

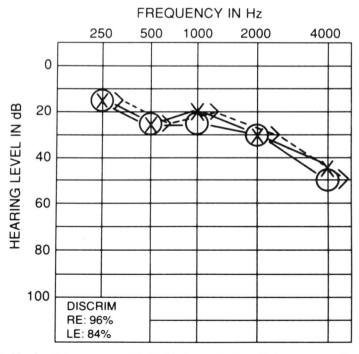

FIG. 23. Audiogram, case 10. M. M. (vascular insufficiency—small vessel disease).

right and 25 dB on the left, with discrimination scores of 96% and 84%, respectively. The ENG was within normal limits (Fig. 24).

The diagnosis of vertigo and unsteadiness secondary to small vessel disease was made, and her medications were adjusted. The patient remained on Persantine. Pavabid and Meclizine were discontinued, and low-dose diazepam therapy (1 mg t.i.d.) was initiated with symptomatic improvement at the 1–3 month follow-up. The patient continued to do well and was returned to the care of her primary physician.

Comment: Older individuals often experience vertigo from vascular insufficiency. Persantine is particularly helpful as it aids circulation by decreasing viscosity of the blood. The authors have found that low-dose diazepam (1 mg) therapy is very helpful in symptomatic relief of the vertigo.

ELECTRONYSTAGMOGRAPHY REPORT

Case 10:   MM

1.   **Spont. Nystagmus** -- _X_ NEG ___ RB ___LB

2.   **Gaze Nystagmus**   -- _X_ NEG ___ RB ___LB

3.   **Optokinetic**   -- _X_ SYM ___ ASYM

4.   **Eye Tracking**   -- ___ I ___ II ___ III ___ IV

5.   **Positionals**   -- ___ NEG ___ RB ___ LB ___ DIR CHG _____

BITHERMAL CALORIC STIMULATION

$R-44^0$	_X_ WNL	___ Slightly Reduced	___ No Response
$L-44^0$	_X_ WNL	___ Slightly Reduced	___ No Response
$R-30^0$	_X_ WNL	___ Slightly Reduced	___ No Response
$L-30^0$	_X_ WNL	___ Slightly Reduced	___ No Response
	_13_ %	_LT_ Unilateral Weakness	
	_13_ %	_RT_ Directional Preponderance	

COMMENT: All caloric responses are within normal limits.

CLINICAL IMPRESSION: Essentially normal recording.

FIG. 24. Electronystagmography (ENG), case 10. M. M. (vascular insufficiency—small vessel disease).

CASE 11.   BENIGN POSITIONAL VERTIGO (BPV)

J.M., a 76-year-old man, presented in May of 1989 with a 10-year history of vertigo occurring only when turning over in bed to the right side with associated nausea and vomiting. He denied tinnitus or fullness in the ears, and there was no fluctuation of hearing. The patient had worn a hearing aid for several years on the right due to a moderate sensorineural hearing loss that had been slowly progressive. There was a strong maternal family history of severe developmental hearing loss; both his mother and grandmother had become deaf late in life. The patient had been placed on Persantine and scopolamine patches as well as a low-salt diet for his symptoms.

The physical exam was within normal limits.

An audiogram showed an SRT of 35 dB on the right with 80% discrimination. On the left the SRT was 20 dB with 84% discrimination (Fig. 25).

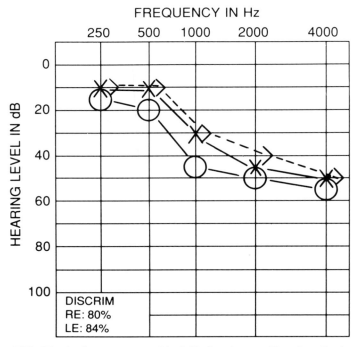

FIG. 25. Audiogram, case 11. J. M. (benign positional vertigo).

The ENG was significant for reduced left vestibular function on cold caloric evaluation (Fig. 26).

There were no abnormalities of the internal auditory canal and cerebellopontine angle (Fig. 27).

The patient was treated with diazepam 5 mg at bedtime, which controlled his symptoms.

Comment: Recently Hismanal (astemizole) has been used successfully in treating BPV. In patients who have their symptoms only when they go to bed, Valium about 1 hour before retiring works very well to control the vertigo.

ELECTRONYSTAGMOGRAPHY REPORT

Case 11:   JM

1.   **Spont. Nystagmus** -- _X_ NEG ___ RB ___LB

2.   **Gaze Nystagmus**   -- _X_ NEG ___ RB ___LB

3.   **Optokinetic**   -- _X_ SYM ___ ASYM

4.   **Eye Tracking**   -- _X_ I ___ II ___ III ___ IV

5.   **Positionals**   -- _X_ NEG ___ RB ___ LB ___ DIR CHG _____

BITHERMAL CALORIC STIMULATION

R-44°	_X_ WNL	___ Slightly Reduced	___ No Response
L-44°	___ WNL	_X_ Slightly Reduced	___ No Response
R-30°	___ WNL	_X_ Slightly Reduced	___ No Response
L-30°	___ WNL	_X_ Slightly Reduced	___ No Response
	_25_ %	_LT_ Unilateral Weakness	
	_1_ %	_LT_ Directional Preponderance	

COMMENT: Caloric responses consistent with left unilateral weakness with no spontaneous or positional nystagmus.

CLINICAL IMPRESSION: Reduced vestibular response, left.

FIG. 26. Electronystagmography (ENG), case 11. J. M. (benign positional vertigo).

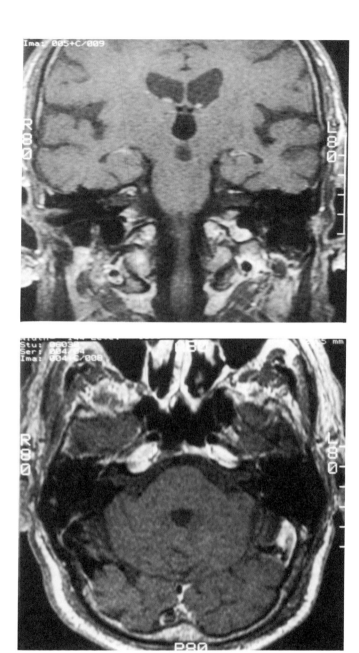

FIG. 27. A: MRI, normal coronal view of internal auditory canals, case 11. J. M. **B:** MRI, normal axial view of internal auditory canals, case 11. J. M.

CASE 12.   PERILYMPH FISTULA

F.H. is a 48-year-old man who presented in April 1984 with a 2½ year history of severe vertiginous episodes occurring every 3 to 6 weeks and lasting for several days. He complained of fullness, tinnitus, and fluctuation all on the right. The initial episodes occurred after a reported skull fracture while playing racquetball with a subsequent 12-hour loss of consciousness.

The physical examination was within normal limits except for a weakly positive right fistula test.

An audiogram showed an SRT of 10 dB with 88% discrimination on the right. The SRT on the left was 0 with 100% discrimination. (Fig. 28). The ENG showed a right-beating positional nystagmus.

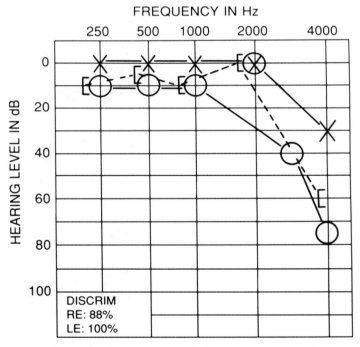

FIG. 28. Audiogram, case 12. F. H. (perilymph fistula).

(Fig. 29). An ABR was within normal limits bilaterally (Fig. 30).

The diagnosis of a perilymph fistula was entertained because of the history of trauma. An exploratory tympanotomy was performed and revealed a disarticulated incudostapedial joint that transmitted normally as evidenced by the preop audiogram. There was cogenital dehiscence of the facial nerve and a fracture of the footplate of the stapes with a perilymph leak. The oval and round windows were patched with fat grafts from the lobule. He had an uneventful postoperative course with resolution of symptoms, and long-term follow-up indicates he has had no further vertigo.

Comment: Head trauma followed by vertigo should make one suspicious of a fistula. Exploration is the most reliable method of establishing the diagnosis.

ELECTRONYSTAGMOGRAPHY REPORT

Case 12: FH

1. **Spont. Nystagmus** -- ___ NEG ___ RB _X_ LB

2. **Gaze Nystagmus** -- _X_ NEG ___ RB ___ LB

3. **Optokinetic** -- _X_ SYM ___ ASYM

4. **Eye Tracking** -- ___ I _X_ II ___ III ___ IV

5. **Positionals** -- ___ NEG ___ RB _X_ LB ___ DIR CHG HF;HBL;LL

BITHERMAL CALORIC STIMULATION

R-44°	_X_ WNL	___ Slightly Reduced	___ No Response
L-44°	_X_ WNL	___ Slightly Reduced	___ No Response
R-30°	_X_ WNL	___ Slightly Reduced	___ No Response
L-30°	_X_ WNL	___ Slightly Reduced	___ No Response
	_____ %	_____ Unilateral Weakness	
	_____ %	_____ Directional Preponderance	

COMMENT: Insignificant left unilateral weakness.

CLINICAL IMPRESSION: Abnormal recording. (Left beating positional nystagmus).

FIG. 29. Electronystagmography (ENG), case 12. F. H. (perilymph fistula).

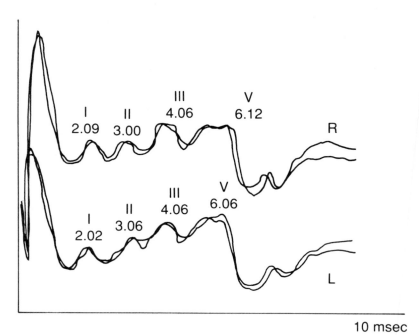

FIG. 30. Auditory brainstem response (ABR), case 12. F. H. (perilymph fistula).

CASE 13. ABNORMAL DILANTIN LEVEL

B.D., a 53-year-old man, presented in January 1989 with increasing vertigo, unsteadiness, and bilateral tinnitus over the previous few weeks.

The patient's past medical history was significant for a 19-year history of well-controlled epilepsy. Current medications included phenobarbital 60 mg at bedtime and Dilantin (phenytoin sodium) 400 mg daily. He had previously been noted to have rotatory nystagmus with a down-beating component.

The physical examination was within normal limits.

An audiogram showed an SRT of 15 dB with 96% discrimination on the right and an SRT of 10 dB with 100% discrimination on the left (Fig. 31).

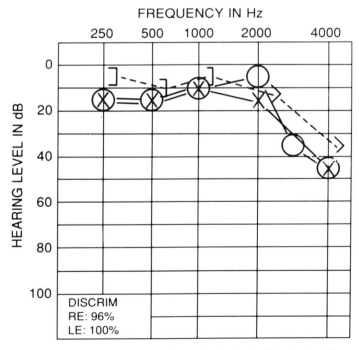

FIG. 31. Audiogram, case 13. B. D. (toxic dilantin level).

The ABR was within normal limits bilaterally (Fig. 32).

An ENG showed symmetric optokinetic but reduced vestibular response on the left to caloric stimuli (Fig. 33).

An MRI was within normal limits. Dilantin levels were obtained and reported to be 28.6 mcg/ml. The upper level of normal is 20 mcg/ml.

The patient's Dilantin was decreased, and Xanax was added on an as-needed basis with improvement of his symptoms.

Comment: Medicines have side effects and toxic levels. Any vertiginous patient who is on regular medications could be experiencing a toxic reaction. Dilantin is notorious for producing vertigo and disequilibrium at toxic levels. Treatment consists of lowering the dosage.

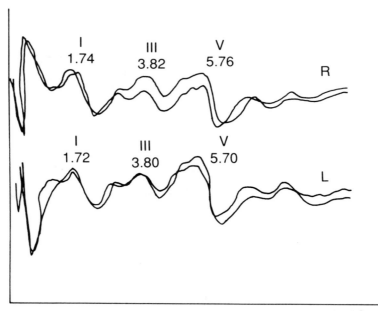

10 msec

FIG. 32. Auditory brainstem response (ABR), case 13. B. D. (toxic Dilantin level).

ELECTRONYSTAGMOGRAPHY REPORT

Case 13: BD

1. **Spont. Nystagmus** -- _X_ NEG ___ RB ___LB

2. **Gaze Nystagmus** -- _X_ NEG ___ RB ___LB

3. **Optokinetic** -- ___ SYM _X_ ASYM

4. **Eye Tracking** -- _X_ I ___ II ___ III ___ IV

5. **Positionals** -- _X_ NEG ___ RB ___ LB ___ DIR CHG ___

BITHERMAL CALORIC STIMULATION

R-44^0 _X_ WNL ___ Slightly Reduced ___ No Response

L-44^0 ___ WNL ___ Slightly Reduced _X_ No Response

R-30^0 _X_ WNL ___ Slightly Reduced ___ No Response

L-30^0 ___ WNL ___ Slightly Reduced _X_ No Response

_100_ % _LT_ Unilateral Weakness

_23_ % _RT_ Directional Preponderance

COMMENT: Caloric stimulation shows left unilateral weakness with no spontaneous or positional nystagmus.

CLINICAL IMPRESSION: Reduced vestibular response, left.

FIG. 33. Electronystagmography (ENG), case 13. B. D. (toxic Dilantin level).

CASE 14.   CEREBELLAR INFARCTION

G.K., a 52-year-old white woman, presented in August 1989 with complaints of constant slow spinning vertigo without hearing changes or tinnitus. Four weeks prior to evaluation she had experienced initial acute vertiginous episodes and a brief loss of consciousness. After arousal she continued to be vertiginous with nausea and vomiting, was unable to speak coherently, and noticed poor coordination of her extremities. All symptoms resolved within 1 hour except that of vertigo. An MRI scan was obtained that showed a small cerebellar infarction.

On physical examination 4 weeks after the onset of symptoms there was mild jerking of the right eye on extraocular movement. Slight decreased right corneal sensation was also present. The remainder of the examination was normal.

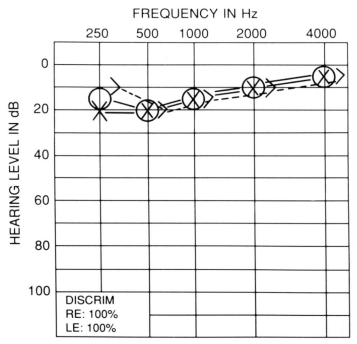

FIG. 34. Audiogram, case 14. G. K. (cerebellar infarction).

The audiogram was normal (Fig. 34) with SRTs of 15 dB and discrimination scores of 100% bilaterally. The ENG was within normal limits.

Treatment of the cerebellar infarction has been supportive. It was felt that an inner ear process did not contribute to the patient's symptoms.

Comment: Loss of consciousness following a vertiginous episode is unusual and generally indicates a central rather than a peripheral lesion. The MRI has literally revolutionized the ability to diagnose a lesion such as this cerebellar infarct.

CASE 15.   TRAUMATIC LABYRINTHITIS—TEMPORAL
BONE FRACTURE

J.M., a 21-year-old man, was seen on October 7, 1982 with a history of falling from a second floor balcony sustaining a transverse basilar skull fracture 7 months prior to referral. The patient was acutely vertiginous for the first 10 days following his injury. Immediately following the injury he experienced a left-sided cerebral spinal otorrhea that subsided spontaneously. An audiogram revealed a left dead ear (Fig. 35).

Labyrinthine sedatives were used in the early stages of his vertiginous episodes. This young man eventually required a tympanoplasty to remove a cholesteatoma from a posterior external auditory canal wall fracture.

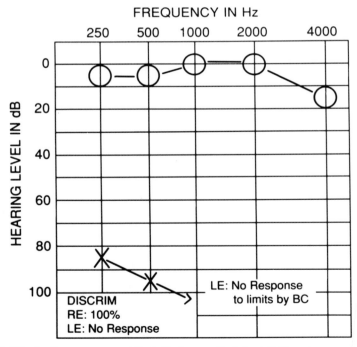

FIG. 35. Audiogram, case 15. J. M. (traumatic labyrinthitis—temporal bone fracture).

Comment: A transverse fracture through the labyrinth usually results in a dead ear and a loss of vestibular function. The vertiginous symptoms are similar to those experienced by an individual undergoing a labyrinthectomy. Once the acute phase has subsided, a period of disequilibrium follows. When compensation occurs the disequilibrium subsides.

ACKNOWLEDGMENT

Chris Johnson, MD, assisted in the preparation of case histories for this chapter.

Subject Index

A

Acoustic neuromas, 38, 41,
    48–49
    case study of, 73–75, *73–75*
Alprazolam, 52
Ampullae, 2
Angiography, cerebral, 46
Anterior inferior cerebellar artery
    (AICA), 47
Anticholinergics, 52
Anticoagulants, 56
Antihistamines, 52
Antivert, 52
Arcus senilis, 18
Arteriograms, *87, 88*
Aspirin, 56
Astemizole, 55
Astrocytomas, 49
Ataxia, 20, 47, 48, 54
Atherosclerotic vascular disease,
    lacunar syndrome in, 48
Audiograms
    in case studies, *64, 66, 69, 73,
    76, 79, 82, 84, 86, 89, 91,
    94, 97, 100, 102*
    in Meniere's disease, 37, *64, 66*
Audiometry, 23
Auditory brainstem response
    (ABR) testing, 23–25, *24,*
    32, 49, 59, *68, 71, 74, 77,
    80, 83, 98*

Aura, in posterior fossa migraine,
    46
Auricle, clinical examination
    of, 15
Autoimmune vestibulopathy, 42
    medical management of, 55–56

B

Balance, three sensory inputs
    responsible for, 31
Barony noise box, 16
Barotrauma, 41
Bekesey audiometry, 23
Benadryl, 52, 53
Benign paroxysmal positional ver-
    tigo (BPPV), 23, 40–41
    medical management of, 55
    surgical management of, 60
Benign positional vertigo (BPV),
    case study of, 91–93,
    91, 93
Benzodiazepines, 52
BERA, in Meniere's disease, 37
Beta-blockers, 56
Bilateral vestibular ablation,
    54, 56
Blood pressure, 15
Blood tests, 32
Bony labyrinth, *2*
    membranous labyrinth with, *3*

Note: References to illustrations are in *italics*.